Hydrocephalus and Mental Health

Hydrocephalus and Mental Health

Matthew Petchinsky

1

Hydrocephalus and Mental Health

By: Matthew Petchinsky

Disclaimer

This book is intended to provide educational information, emotional encouragement, and supportive reflections for individuals living with hydrocephalus and the many mental and emotional experiences that may accompany the condition. Living with hydrocephalus can affect many areas of life—including energy levels, cognition, emotional stability, stress tolerance, and daily functioning—and the purpose of this book is to offer understanding, perspective, and practical ideas that may help readers navigate those challenges with greater resilience. The insights, reflections, and strategies presented throughout this book are designed to support personal growth, self-awareness, and emotional strength, but they are not meant to diagnose, treat, cure, or prevent any medical or psychological condition.

The information in this book should not be considered medical advice, mental health treatment, or a replacement for care from qualified healthcare professionals. Hydrocephalus is a complex neurological condition that often requires ongoing medical monitoring and individualized treatment plans. Readers should always consult with licensed physicians, neurologists, neurosurgeons, psychologists, psychiatrists, or other qualified healthcare providers regarding symptoms, medications, treatments, mental health concerns, or medical decisions related to their condition. Any lifestyle suggestions, emotional coping tools, or reflective exercises included in this book are offered as supportive resources that may complement professional care, not replace it.

Mental health experiences associated with hydrocephalus can vary widely from person to person. Some individuals may face anxiety, depression, fatigue, cognitive strain, memory challenges, or emotional overwhelm due to the physical and neurological impacts of the condition. The discussions in this book are meant to acknowledge those realities and provide compassionate encouragement. However, if readers experience severe emotional distress, persistent depression, suicidal thoughts, neurological changes, worsening symptoms, or any medical emergency, they should immediately seek help from licensed healthcare professionals or emergency medical services.

This book may also discuss lifestyle practices such as mindfulness, stress management, journaling, self-reflection, gentle physical activities, and supportive mindset approaches. These practices are offered as tools for personal empowerment and emotional resilience. Individual results will vary, and readers should use their own judgment and consult healthcare providers when implementing any new routines, particularly if they have shunts, pressure sensitivity, seizures, mobility limitations, or other medical considerations related to hydrocephalus.

Every person's journey with hydrocephalus is unique. What works for one individual may not work the same way for another. Readers are encouraged to approach the ideas in this book with curiosity, patience, and self-compassion, adapting the practices in ways that feel safe and appropriate for their personal circumstances. The author and publisher make no guarantees regarding outcomes and assume no responsibility for how the information in this book is applied.

Ultimately, this book is offered in the spirit of support, understanding, and empowerment. Its goal is to help readers feel less alone, better informed, and more capable of navigating the emotional landscape that can accompany hydrocephalus. Professional medical care, trusted support networks, and ongoing communication with healthcare providers remain essential parts of managing both hydrocephalus and mental well-being.

Introduction

The mind is often compared to water for a reason. Water flows, bends, adapts, and reshapes the landscapes it touches. It can be calm and reflective like a still lake, or powerful and relentless like a rushing river cutting through stone. Our thoughts, emotions, and perceptions move in similar ways—sometimes peaceful, sometimes overwhelming, and often changing from moment to moment.

For individuals living with hydrocephalus, the inner landscape of the mind can feel especially complex. Hydrocephalus is often understood primarily as a neurological condition affecting the brain's fluid balance, yet its effects extend far beyond physical symptoms. The emotional world can shift in subtle or dramatic ways. Some days may feel steady and manageable, while others may bring waves of fatigue, anxiety, confusion, frustration, or self-doubt. These experiences are not signs of weakness; they are natural responses to navigating a condition that influences both the body and the mind.

Many people living with hydrocephalus find themselves walking a path that others may not fully understand. There may be cognitive fatigue that arrives without warning, moments when concentration becomes difficult, or emotional swings that feel confusing and hard to explain. Medical appointments, treatments, and the constant awareness of one's health can also create an ongoing background pressure that affects mental well-being.

Because of this, caring for the mind becomes just as important as caring for the body.

The purpose of this book is not to offer unrealistic promises or quick solutions. Instead, it aims to provide practical tools and thoughtful reflections that can support emotional resilience while living with hydrocephalus. Mental well-being is not about eliminating every difficult thought or emotion. Rather, it involves learning how to move through those experiences with awareness, patience, and compassion for oneself.

Nature offers many powerful lessons in resilience. Rivers carve valleys through mountains over time, not through sudden force but through persistence. Trees bend with the wind rather than breaking. The tides rise and fall in steady rhythms that have existed for millennia. These patterns remind us that strength is not always loud or dramatic. Sometimes strength is quiet endurance, steady adaptation, and the willingness to keep moving forward even when conditions are challenging.

The human mind works in similar ways. While hydrocephalus may create unique mental and emotional challenges, the brain also possesses a remarkable capacity to adapt and reorganize itself. Neuroscience has repeatedly shown that the brain is not fixed; it is capable of learning, adjusting, and forming new pathways throughout life. This concept, known as neuroplasticity, means that supportive habits, emotional awareness, and thoughtful mental practices can gradually shape how we experience stress, frustration, and uncertainty.

Throughout this book, readers will encounter ideas and practices designed to nurture this adaptive capacity. These include approaches such as mindful awareness, emotional grounding, stress regulation, and compassionate self-reflection. None of these practices require perfection. They are simply tools—gentle ways of learning how to observe the mind, calm the nervous system, and build inner steadiness over time.

Mindfulness, for example, is not about emptying the mind of all thoughts. Instead, it is about noticing thoughts and emotions without immediately becoming overwhelmed by them. By learning to pause and observe what is happening internally, individuals can create a small but meaningful space between experience and reaction. Within that space lies the ability to respond with greater clarity and self-understanding.

Emotional grounding practices can also play a powerful role in supporting mental health. Living with a neurological condition can sometimes make life feel unpredictable. Grounding techniques help bring attention back to the present moment, reconnecting the mind with the body and the surrounding environment. Even simple actions—such as focusing on breathing, noticing physical sensations, or writing down thoughts—can provide stability during moments of mental turbulence.

Another important theme of this book is self-compassion. Many individuals living with hydrocephalus place immense pressure on themselves to function in ways that match societal expectations. When energy levels fluctuate or concentration becomes difficult, it can lead to feelings of guilt, frustration, or inadequacy. Yet healing rarely grows from self-criticism. Growth tends to emerge from patience, kindness toward oneself, and the understanding that every person's journey is unique.

Self-compassion does not mean ignoring challenges or pretending everything is easy. Instead, it involves recognizing one's struggles honestly while offering the same understanding and care that we might extend to a friend facing similar difficulties. When individuals begin to treat themselves with this level of gentleness, the mental burden of chronic conditions often becomes more manageable.

Resilience is another central idea explored throughout these pages. Resilience is not about never experiencing stress, sadness, or exhaustion. Those experiences are part of being human, and they are particularly common for people managing long-term health conditions. True resilience is the ability to recover, adjust, and continue moving forward even when life feels difficult.

For many individuals living with hydrocephalus, resilience has already been demonstrated countless times—through surgeries, medical treatments, daily adaptations, and moments of perseverance that may go unnoticed by others. This book seeks to recognize that strength and help readers cultivate even deeper levels of emotional balance and confidence.

Within these chapters, readers will find practical guidance for navigating common mental health challenges associated with hydrocephalus. Topics may include managing anxiety, reducing mental fatigue, strengthening emotional awareness, improving daily coping strategies, and building a supportive internal dialogue. Reflective exercises, journaling prompts, and grounding practices are included to help translate ideas into real-life experiences.

These tools are not meant to be rigid instructions. Instead, they are invitations. Each reader is encouraged to explore them at their own pace, adapting them to fit personal needs, energy levels, and circumstances. Some practices may resonate strongly, while others may feel less relevant. That is perfectly natural. The goal is not perfection, but discovery—finding the approaches that help support your own sense of balance and well-being.

Living with hydrocephalus may bring moments of uncertainty, but it can also reveal deep reservoirs of strength, creativity, and self-awareness. Many individuals who navigate neurological challenges develop a profound understanding of patience, adaptability, and resilience. These qualities can become powerful sources of personal wisdom.

The journey toward mental well-being is rarely a straight line. There will be days of clarity and days of struggle, moments of confidence and moments of doubt. Yet, much like water shaping stone over time, consistent care for the mind gradually creates change.

With awareness, compassion, and supportive practices, the inner landscape can become calmer, steadier, and more resilient.

This book is an invitation to begin—or continue—that journey.

Chapter 1: Understanding Emotional Waves

The Mind as an Emotional Tide

Living with hydrocephalus often means becoming familiar with emotional patterns that may feel unpredictable or overwhelming at times. Many people experience waves of emotion that seem to rise and fall without clear explanation. These emotional tides can include anxiety, sadness, irritability, mental fatigue, or moments of deep frustration. While these feelings can feel confusing, they are often connected to the complex relationship between the brain, the nervous system, and emotional processing.

The brain is not only responsible for thought and movement; it is also the central regulator of mood, perception, and emotional response. When neurological conditions affect the brain, even subtly, emotional experiences can shift as well. Hydrocephalus can influence how the brain processes stress, stimulation, and cognitive effort. Because of this, individuals may notice emotional responses that feel stronger, more sensitive, or more exhausting than expected.

Emotions themselves are not problems to be fixed. They are signals. They communicate information about internal states, external pressures, and the body's response to the environment. Just as ocean tides move with the gravitational pull of the moon, emotions move in response to both internal neurological processes and external life circumstances. Understanding this dynamic can transform frustration into insight.

For many people, the first step toward emotional balance is recognizing that emotional waves are natural. Experiencing fluctuations does not mean something is wrong with you. It simply means your nervous system is responding to a variety of influences—physical, mental, and environmental. Acknowledging this reality can reduce the sense of confusion that often accompanies emotional shifts.

When emotional waves are understood rather than resisted, they often become easier to navigate. Instead of feeling like an uncontrollable storm, they begin to resemble tides that can be observed, anticipated, and gradually managed. This awareness lays the foundation for emotional resilience.

The Neurological Connection to Mood

Hydrocephalus can affect areas of the brain involved in mood regulation, cognitive processing, and stress response. The brain contains networks responsible for emotional regulation, including regions such as the limbic system, the prefrontal cortex, and the hypothalamus. When pressure changes or neurological fatigue occur, these systems may respond differently than they would in someone without neurological challenges.

For some individuals, this may appear as heightened emotional sensitivity. Situations that once felt manageable might suddenly feel overwhelming. Concentration can become more difficult, which may lead to frustration or mental exhaustion. Emotional responses may arise more quickly, sometimes before the mind has time to fully process what is happening.

Neurological fatigue is another common factor influencing mood. When the brain works harder to process information, it can become tired more quickly. This mental fatigue can lead to irritability, emotional exhaustion, or a sense of being mentally overloaded. Understanding that these reactions may have neurological roots can help reduce self-blame.

It is also important to remember that mood is influenced by many factors beyond the neurological condition itself. Sleep quality, physical pain, medications, stress levels, social interactions, and environmental stimuli all interact with brain chemistry. When several of these factors occur simultaneously, emotional intensity can increase.

Recognizing the neurological component of mood does not mean that emotions are purely biological or beyond influence. Instead, it helps explain why certain feelings arise and why self-care strategies—such as rest, mindfulness, and emotional awareness—can play such an important role in maintaining balance.

Recognizing Emotional Fluctuations

Emotional awareness begins with noticing patterns. Many individuals living with hydrocephalus report experiencing cycles of emotional highs and lows that may not initially seem connected to anything specific. Learning to observe these patterns can provide valuable insight into the mind's rhythms.

Some emotional fluctuations may follow predictable triggers. For example, mental fatigue after a long day of concentration may lead to irritability or emotional sensitivity. Overstimulation from noise, bright lights, or social interactions may also create emotional strain. Identifying these triggers can help individuals prepare for and manage emotional shifts.

Other fluctuations may appear more subtle. There may be days when motivation feels low without a clear reason, or moments when anxiety seems to appear suddenly. These experiences can be unsettling, but they often reflect the brain's natural response to accumulated stress or cognitive effort.

Keeping track of emotional patterns can help reveal connections between mood and lifestyle factors. For instance, sleep patterns, hydration, nutrition, and daily stress levels can all influence emotional stability. Over time, individuals may begin to notice relationships between their physical condition and emotional responses.

The goal of recognizing emotional fluctuations is not to eliminate emotions but to understand them. When individuals become familiar with their emotional patterns, they gain the ability to respond more thoughtfully rather than feeling controlled by sudden emotional shifts.

Accepting Feelings Without Judgment

One of the most powerful skills in emotional well-being is learning to experience feelings without immediately judging them. Many people are taught to label certain emotions as "good" or "bad," which can create internal conflict when difficult feelings arise. For someone living with hydrocephalus, this judgment can intensify emotional stress.

Feelings such as frustration, sadness, fear, or exhaustion are not personal failures. They are natural responses to challenging circumstances. When individuals attempt to suppress or ignore these emotions, the mind often becomes more tense. The energy required to push emotions away can increase mental fatigue.

Acceptance does not mean giving up or resigning oneself to suffering. Instead, it means allowing emotions to be present without fighting them. When emotions are acknowledged with curiosity rather than criticism, they often become less overwhelming. This approach allows individuals to observe feelings as temporary experiences rather than permanent states.

Practicing emotional acceptance can create a sense of inner calm. Instead of feeling trapped in emotional reactions, individuals begin to develop a more balanced relationship with their thoughts and feelings. Over time, this mindset can reduce stress and promote emotional stability.

Learning to say, "This is how I feel right now, and that is okay," can be surprisingly powerful. This simple shift in perspective creates space for healing and self-understanding.

The Role of Stress in Neurological Health

Stress has a profound influence on both mental and physical well-being. For individuals living with hydrocephalus, stress can amplify existing neurological challenges. When the body enters a state of stress, it activates the nervous system's survival mechanisms, releasing hormones such as cortisol and adrenaline.

These stress responses are useful in short bursts, helping the body react quickly to danger or pressure. However, when stress becomes chronic, it can strain the nervous system. Prolonged stress may lead to increased mental fatigue, irritability, sleep disruption, and difficulty concentrating.

Neurological conditions can make the brain more sensitive to stress triggers. Situations that might seem minor to others—such as noise, time pressure, or crowded environments—may feel overwhelming. This heightened sensitivity is not a weakness but a reflection of how the brain processes stimuli.

Managing stress becomes an important part of protecting neurological health. Simple practices such as rest, breathing exercises, mindful pauses, and balanced daily routines can help regulate the nervous system. These practices encourage the body to move out of survival mode and return to a calmer state.

When individuals learn to recognize stress signals early, they gain the opportunity to respond before stress becomes overwhelming. This awareness is one of the most valuable tools for maintaining emotional stability.

Learning Emotional Self-Awareness

Emotional self-awareness is the ability to recognize and understand what one is feeling in the present moment. This skill allows individuals to observe emotions without becoming immediately overwhelmed by them. For people living with hydrocephalus, developing this awareness can create greater control over emotional responses.

Self-awareness begins with curiosity. Instead of asking "Why am I like this?" a more helpful question may be "What am I feeling right now?" This shift moves the focus from self-criticism to exploration. By noticing emotional states without judgment, individuals can better understand their internal experiences.

Over time, emotional self-awareness can reveal patterns. Certain environments may trigger stress, while certain activities may create calm. Some individuals discover that quiet reflection helps restore balance, while others benefit from gentle movement or creative expression.

Building emotional awareness also strengthens communication. When individuals understand their emotional needs, they can express those needs more clearly to others. This can improve relationships, reduce misunderstandings, and create stronger support systems.

Emotional self-awareness is not developed overnight. It grows gradually through practice and reflection. Each moment of noticing an emotion—whether calm or difficult—is a step toward greater understanding and resilience.

Exercises

Exercise 1: Emotional Weather Mapping

Step 1: At the end of each day, pause and reflect on your emotional experiences throughout the day.

Step 2: Imagine your emotions as different types of weather—sunny, cloudy, stormy, windy, or calm.

Step 3: Write down which "weather pattern" best describes your emotional state during different parts of the day.

Step 4: Note any events, activities, or physical sensations that may have influenced these emotional changes.

Step 5: Review your notes after several days to see if patterns begin to appear.

Exercise 2: The Pause and Name Method

Step 1: When you notice a strong emotion, pause for a moment instead of reacting immediately.

Step 2: Take three slow breaths, allowing your body to relax slightly.

Step 3: Identify the emotion you are experiencing and name it silently or aloud.

Step 4: Remind yourself that emotions are temporary and will shift with time.

Step 5: Choose a calm response instead of reacting automatically.

Exercise 3: Body Awareness Grounding

Step 1: Sit comfortably and close your eyes if it feels safe to do so.

Step 2: Slowly bring your attention to different parts of your body, starting at your feet and moving upward.

Step 3: Notice any sensations such as tension, warmth, or relaxation.

Step 4: Take slow breaths while imagining tension leaving your body.

Step 5: After several minutes, gently open your eyes and observe how your emotional state has shifted.

Journal Prompts

1. What emotions do I experience most frequently throughout the week?
2. When do I feel the most emotionally calm?
3. What situations tend to trigger stress or frustration?
4. How does fatigue affect my emotional state?
5. What physical sensations accompany my emotions?
6. What activities help restore emotional balance?
7. How do I usually respond when difficult emotions appear?
8. What would it look like to treat my emotions with compassion?
9. What patterns am I beginning to notice in my emotional waves?
10. What small change could help me support my emotional well-being?

Closing Reflection

Emotions are not obstacles on the path of healing; they are part of the journey itself. Living with hydrocephalus may bring emotional waves that feel powerful or confusing at times, yet those waves also carry valuable information about the mind and body. When we learn to observe emotions rather than resist them, we gain the ability to navigate life with greater awareness and balance.

Understanding emotional patterns is the first step toward emotional resilience. Through patience, curiosity, and compassionate self-awareness, individuals can learn to ride the tides of emotion rather than being overwhelmed by them.

Like water shaping the shoreline over time, small moments of awareness gradually transform the inner landscape. Each step toward understanding brings greater calm, clarity, and strength.

Chapter 2: Anxiety and the Flow of Thought

Understanding the Nature of Anxiety

Anxiety is one of the most common emotional experiences for individuals living with neurological conditions such as hydrocephalus. The brain is responsible for monitoring the body and environment for potential threats, and when the nervous system becomes overwhelmed or fatigued, it can become more sensitive to signals of stress. This heightened sensitivity may lead to frequent worry, racing thoughts, physical tension, or sudden feelings of panic.

For some individuals, anxiety may appear gradually throughout the day. Small pressures accumulate—mental fatigue, unexpected disruptions, or cognitive overload—until the mind begins to feel crowded with worry. For others, anxiety may arise suddenly, seemingly without warning. The body may react with a racing heart, shallow breathing, dizziness, or a sense of losing control.

It is important to understand that anxiety is not a character flaw. It is a protective mechanism built into the human nervous system. The brain is constantly evaluating whether a situation feels safe or unsafe. When the brain perceives uncertainty, it activates a cascade of signals designed to prepare the body for action.

However, when the nervous system remains in a heightened state of alert for long periods of time, anxiety can become exhausting. Individuals living with hydrocephalus may already experience neurological fatigue, making prolonged stress responses particularly draining. Learning how anxiety functions is the first step toward managing it with greater awareness and calm.

When anxiety is understood rather than feared, it begins to lose some of its power. Recognizing anxiety as a signal rather than a threat allows individuals to respond with supportive strategies that calm the mind and restore balance.

Recognizing Anxiety Triggers

Every person experiences anxiety differently, and the triggers that activate anxious thoughts can vary widely. For individuals managing hydrocephalus, triggers may include cognitive fatigue, overstimulation, sudden changes in routine, physical discomfort, or worries about health and daily functioning.

Environmental factors can also play a significant role. Loud environments, bright lights, crowded spaces, or long periods of concentration may place additional strain on the nervous system. When the brain is already working harder to process information, these conditions can push mental stress beyond comfortable limits.

Emotional triggers may also arise from uncertainty or fear about the future. Living with a neurological condition can create understandable concerns about health stability, independence, or personal goals. When these thoughts circulate repeatedly in the mind, they can gradually build into anxiety.

Recognizing triggers does not mean eliminating them completely. Life inevitably includes stressors and uncertainties. Instead, the goal is to become familiar with the patterns that tend to precede anxious feelings. Awareness allows individuals to anticipate stress responses and apply calming strategies before anxiety escalates.

Over time, identifying triggers can transform anxiety from a mysterious force into a recognizable pattern. This knowledge provides a sense of control and allows individuals to respond with intention rather than reaction.

Grounding the Mind During Panic

When anxiety intensifies into panic, the body's survival system becomes highly activated. The heart may race, breathing may become shallow, and thoughts may spiral rapidly. In these moments, the nervous system is attempting to protect the body from perceived danger.

Grounding techniques help interrupt this cycle by gently bringing attention back to the present moment. These practices signal to the nervous system that immediate danger is not present, allowing the body to gradually return to a calmer state.

One effective grounding strategy involves focusing attention on the senses. Noticing the feel of the floor beneath your feet, the sound of nearby objects, or the sensation of air moving through the lungs can help redirect the mind away from spiraling thoughts.

Slow breathing also plays a powerful role in calming panic. When the breath becomes slower and deeper, it activates the parasympathetic nervous system, which helps the body shift out of its stress response. Even a few minutes of controlled breathing can reduce the intensity of panic symptoms.

Grounding techniques do not eliminate anxiety instantly, but they provide a pathway back to stability. With practice, these techniques can become reliable tools that restore emotional balance during moments of distress.

Slowing the River of Racing Thoughts

Anxiety often feels like a river moving too quickly for the mind to follow. Thoughts may jump from one worry to another, creating a sense of mental chaos. This rapid thinking can make it difficult to concentrate, relax, or make decisions.

Racing thoughts frequently arise when the brain attempts to solve multiple problems simultaneously. The mind becomes trapped in a loop of "what if" scenarios, constantly searching for solutions or predicting potential dangers. While the brain believes it is helping, this process often increases stress rather than reducing it.

Slowing this mental river begins with recognizing that not every thought requires immediate attention. Thoughts are mental events, not commands. Learning to observe thoughts without immediately reacting to them can create valuable space between worry and response.

Mindfulness practices are particularly helpful in slowing racing thoughts. By focusing attention on breathing, physical sensations, or simple tasks, individuals can gently guide the mind away from anxious spirals. This practice does not suppress thoughts; instead, it allows them to pass through awareness without dominating it.

Over time, individuals may discover that racing thoughts lose intensity when they are observed calmly rather than resisted. The mind begins to settle, much like water calming after a storm.

Creating Calming Daily Rituals

Rituals provide structure and predictability, which can be deeply comforting for the nervous system. When daily life feels uncertain or overwhelming, consistent routines create small islands of stability throughout the day.

Calming rituals do not need to be complicated or time-consuming. Simple practices such as drinking tea quietly in the morning, taking a short walk, stretching gently, or spending a few minutes journaling can signal to the brain that it is safe to relax.

For individuals living with hydrocephalus, rituals can also support neurological recovery. Scheduled rest periods, quiet reflection, or mindful breathing breaks can reduce cognitive fatigue and prevent stress from building throughout the day.

Rituals also create psychological boundaries between different parts of the day. A morning ritual may help ease the transition from sleep to activity, while an evening ritual can signal the mind that it is time to slow down and prepare for rest.

When calming rituals are practiced consistently, they gradually train the nervous system to recognize moments of peace. These moments accumulate over time, strengthening emotional resilience and reducing the frequency of anxiety.

Building Emotional Safety

Emotional safety is the sense that one's internal world is stable, supported, and protected. It does not mean that life is free from challenges. Instead, it means that individuals feel capable of navigating those challenges without losing their sense of balance.

For people living with hydrocephalus, building emotional safety may involve creating environments that reduce stress and encourage calm. This might include organizing living spaces to minimize overstimulation, establishing supportive routines, or surrounding oneself with compassionate relationships.

Internal dialogue also plays an important role in emotional safety. The way individuals speak to themselves during moments of difficulty can either intensify anxiety or provide reassurance. Replacing harsh self-criticism with gentle encouragement can significantly reduce emotional strain.

Support systems are another vital component of emotional safety. Friends, family members, healthcare providers, and supportive communities can provide understanding and reassurance during challenging moments. Knowing that support is available can greatly reduce feelings of isolation.

Ultimately, emotional safety is built through many small acts of care—rest, reflection, supportive relationships, and self-compassion. These practices create a foundation of stability that allows individuals to face anxiety with greater confidence and resilience.

Exercises

Exercise 1: The 5–4–3–2–1 Grounding Method

Step 1: Pause and take a slow breath.

Step 2: Identify **five things** you can see around you.

Step 3: Identify **four things** you can touch.

Step 4: Identify **three things** you can hear.

Step 5: Identify **two things** you can smell and **one thing** you can taste or imagine tasting.

This exercise helps anchor the mind in the present moment and interrupts anxious thought loops.

Exercise 2: The Slow Breath Reset

Step 1: Sit comfortably and place one hand on your abdomen.

Step 2: Inhale slowly through your nose for four seconds.

Step 3: Hold the breath gently for two seconds.

Step 4: Exhale slowly through your mouth for six seconds.

Step 5: Repeat this breathing cycle for five minutes while focusing on the sensation of breath moving through your body.

Exercise 3: The Thought Release Practice

Step 1: Write down the anxious thoughts currently circulating in your mind.

Step 2: Look at each thought and ask yourself whether it represents a real problem that requires action.

Step 3: If the thought requires action, write one small step you can take.

Step 4: If the thought is simply worry, acknowledge it and imagine placing it in a mental container for later reflection.

Step 5: Take three slow breaths and return your attention to the present moment.

Journal Prompts

1. What situations tend to trigger my anxiety most frequently?
2. How does anxiety feel physically in my body?
3. What thoughts tend to appear during moments of panic?
4. What calming practices have helped me before?
5. When do I feel the safest emotionally?
6. What environments make my mind feel peaceful?
7. How can I create small rituals that support calmness?
8. What supportive words can I offer myself during anxiety?
9. What patterns have I noticed in my anxious thoughts?
10. What does emotional safety mean to me?

Closing Reflection

Anxiety can feel like a powerful current pulling the mind in many directions at once. Yet beneath that current lies the steady rhythm of the breath, the grounding presence of the body, and the quiet strength of awareness.

By understanding anxiety triggers, practicing grounding techniques, and creating calming rituals, individuals can learn to navigate anxious moments with greater confidence. The mind may still experience waves of worry, but those waves no longer need to control the entire landscape.

Emotional safety grows slowly through repeated acts of care and awareness. Each moment of calm breathing, each grounding exercise, and each compassionate thought toward oneself strengthens the foundation of resilience.

Like a river that eventually finds its way back to calm waters, the mind also has the ability to return to balance. With patience and practice, anxiety becomes not a permanent storm but a passing current within the larger flow of life.

Chapter 3: Depression and Inner Darkness

Recognizing the Landscape of Depression

Depression can feel like a heavy fog that settles slowly over the mind. For individuals living with hydrocephalus, emotional lows may sometimes appear alongside physical fatigue, neurological strain, or prolonged stress. These emotional states can feel isolating and confusing, particularly when the world continues moving at a pace that feels difficult to match.

Depression is not simply sadness. It can involve a deep loss of energy, motivation, and emotional warmth. Activities that once felt meaningful may begin to feel distant or exhausting. The mind may become quiet and withdrawn, or it may fill with self-critical thoughts that seem difficult to silence.

Many individuals with neurological conditions experience depressive cycles rather than constant depression. There may be periods when mood improves and energy returns, followed by times when emotional heaviness settles in again. These cycles can be influenced by sleep patterns, physical health, stress levels, and neurological fatigue.

Understanding depression as a cycle rather than a permanent state can provide an important shift in perspective. Emotional darkness may feel overwhelming when it arrives, but cycles by nature are temporary. Just as night eventually gives way to morning, depressive states often shift with time, care, and support.

Recognizing the signs of depression early—such as loss of motivation, persistent fatigue, emotional numbness, or increased isolation—can help individuals respond with supportive practices before the cycle deepens.

Understanding Depressive Cycles

Depressive cycles often develop gradually. They may begin with subtle changes in energy, such as increased tiredness or reduced interest in daily activities. Over time, these small shifts can accumulate into a deeper emotional heaviness that affects thinking, motivation, and outlook.

For individuals living with hydrocephalus, neurological fatigue can play a significant role in these cycles. When the brain is under physical or cognitive strain, emotional resilience may decrease. Tasks that normally feel manageable may begin to feel overwhelming, leading to withdrawal or discouragement.

Thought patterns also influence depressive cycles. The mind may begin repeating narratives such as "I'm not doing enough," "I'll never feel better," or "Things will always be this difficult." These thoughts are powerful because they shape how the brain interprets experiences.

It is important to remember that depressive thoughts are not always accurate reflections of reality. They are often expressions of the mind's exhaustion rather than objective truth. Learning to recognize these thoughts as temporary mental states can weaken their influence.

Breaking depressive cycles rarely happens through one dramatic change. Instead, small supportive actions—rest, connection, movement, or creative expression—gradually help the mind shift out of emotional stagnation.

Restoring Hope Through Small Actions

When depression is present, large goals can feel impossible. Even simple tasks may require enormous effort. This is why recovery often begins with very small actions rather than major life changes.

A small action might be something as simple as opening a window, stepping outside for fresh air, writing a few sentences in a journal, or preparing a nourishing meal. These actions may seem insignificant, yet they signal to the mind that movement and care are still possible.

Each small action gently disrupts the inertia that depression creates. The brain begins to receive signals that life continues to move forward, even if progress feels slow. Over time, these small acts accumulate and begin to rebuild momentum.

Hope does not usually appear suddenly. Instead, it grows gradually through repeated moments of effort and self-care. Every small step becomes evidence that change is possible.

For individuals living with hydrocephalus, honoring energy limitations is also important. Small actions should be realistic and sustainable rather than exhausting. The goal is not perfection but gentle forward movement.

Nature as a Source of Emotional Restoration

Nature has long been recognized as a powerful source of emotional healing. Spending time outdoors can calm the nervous system, reduce stress hormones, and improve mood. Even brief contact with natural environments can help restore mental balance.

Natural spaces offer a rhythm that contrasts with the pressures of modern life. Trees grow slowly, rivers flow steadily, and seasons change with patience. Observing these rhythms can remind the mind that change is a natural part of life.

For individuals experiencing depression, nature can provide a quiet sense of connection that does not require conversation or performance. Sitting beneath a tree, feeling sunlight on the skin, or listening to the sound of wind moving through leaves can bring subtle emotional relief.

Nature also encourages sensory awareness. The smell of fresh air, the texture of soil or grass, and the colors of plants can gently pull attention away from heavy thoughts and back into the present moment.

These experiences do not eliminate depression entirely, but they can create small openings of calm and perspective within the emotional landscape.

The Strength of Community Support

Isolation often deepens depressive feelings. When individuals withdraw from others, the mind may begin to believe that support is unavailable or that one must face challenges alone. In reality, connection is one of the most powerful protective factors against depression.

Community support does not always mean large social gatherings. It can be as simple as a trusted friend, a supportive family member, an understanding healthcare provider, or an online group of individuals facing similar challenges.

For people living with hydrocephalus, connecting with others who understand the condition can be particularly valuable. Shared experiences reduce the sense of being misunderstood or alone.

Community also offers practical support. Others may help with daily tasks, provide encouragement, or simply listen without judgment. These interactions remind the mind that challenges are shared rather than faced in isolation.

Allowing oneself to receive support can be difficult, especially for individuals who feel pressure to remain strong. Yet accepting help is not weakness. It is a recognition that human beings are meant to navigate life together.

Cultivating Patience With Oneself

Recovery from depression is rarely immediate. Emotional healing unfolds gradually, often through a process of trial, learning, and self-discovery. Patience becomes an essential companion on this journey.

Many individuals living with hydrocephalus already face significant physical and neurological challenges. Expecting constant productivity or emotional stability under these conditions can create unrealistic pressure.

Self-patience involves acknowledging limitations without self-judgment. Some days will contain energy and motivation, while others may require rest and quiet reflection. Both experiences are valid parts of the healing process.

Compassion toward oneself also means recognizing that emotional struggles do not diminish personal worth. Depression may cloud perception, but it does not erase the strength and resilience that individuals have already demonstrated.

Over time, patience allows emotional wounds to soften and new perspectives to emerge. Healing may move slowly, but every moment of self-understanding contributes to the journey forward.

Exercises

Exercise 1: The One Small Step Practice

Step 1: Choose one small action that feels manageable today.

Step 2: Write down the action before completing it.

Step 3: Complete the action slowly and mindfully.

Step 4: After finishing, acknowledge the effort you made.

Step 5: Record how you feel emotionally after completing the task.

Repeat this process daily to build gradual momentum.

Exercise 2: Nature Reconnection Practice

Step 1: Find a quiet natural space such as a park, garden, or shaded outdoor area.

Step 2: Sit comfortably and focus on your breathing for a few moments.

Step 3: Observe your surroundings using your senses—notice sounds, colors, textures, and scents.

Step 4: Allow your thoughts to slow as you observe the natural environment.

Step 5: Spend at least ten minutes simply experiencing the presence of nature.

Exercise 3: Compassionate Self-Talk

Step 1: Write down a negative thought you often experience during difficult moments.

Step 2: Reflect on how you would respond if a friend expressed the same thought.

Step 3: Rewrite the thought as a compassionate message to yourself.

Step 4: Read the compassionate message aloud or silently.

Step 5: Repeat this practice whenever self-critical thoughts arise.

Journal Prompts

1. What signs tell me that I may be entering a depressive cycle?
2. What small actions help me feel even slightly better during difficult days?
3. How does nature affect my mood and mental clarity?
4. Who are the supportive people in my life?
5. What makes it difficult for me to ask for help?
6. What thoughts tend to appear during depressive periods?
7. What would self-compassion look like in my daily life?
8. What activities once brought me peace or joy?
9. How can I create small moments of hope each day?
10. What strengths have helped me navigate past emotional challenges?

Closing Reflection

Depression can feel like walking through a long night without knowing when morning will arrive. Yet even the darkest night contains the quiet promise of dawn. Emotional darkness does not last forever, even when it feels endless.

By recognizing depressive cycles, taking small steps toward hope, reconnecting with nature, and seeking support from others, individuals can gradually rediscover light within the mind. Each moment of care—no matter how small—contributes to healing.

Patience and compassion toward oneself are essential companions on this journey. Healing rarely happens quickly, but every step forward, every breath of fresh air, and every supportive connection reminds us that the mind is capable of renewal.

Even within darkness, the seeds of light remain present, waiting patiently for the moment they can grow again.

Chapter 4: Self-Compassion and Inner Healing

Understanding the Power of Self-Compassion

Self-compassion is one of the most transformative tools available for emotional healing. For many individuals living with hydrocephalus, life has involved navigating physical limitations, medical challenges, fatigue, and emotional uncertainty. These experiences can sometimes lead to harsh self-judgment, where the mind quietly whispers that one should be stronger, faster, or more capable than current circumstances allow.

Yet healing rarely grows from criticism. When the mind constantly attacks itself with blame or disappointment, emotional energy becomes trapped in a cycle of tension and discouragement. Over time, this pattern can deepen feelings of exhaustion and sadness. Self-compassion offers a different path—one rooted in patience, understanding, and kindness toward one's own struggles.

Self-compassion does not mean ignoring challenges or pretending that everything is easy. Instead, it means recognizing the reality of difficulty while responding to oneself with care rather than punishment. It is the same type of kindness we naturally extend to friends or loved ones when they face hardship.

For individuals managing neurological conditions, self-compassion becomes especially important. The body and brain may require more rest, more recovery time, and more flexibility than others might expect. When this reality is accepted with gentleness rather than frustration, the mind becomes a supportive ally rather than an internal critic.

Learning self-compassion is not a single decision but a gradual practice. Each moment of kindness toward oneself creates a new pattern in the mind, slowly replacing old habits of self-judgment with understanding.

Letting Go of Self-Blame

Many people living with chronic conditions carry hidden burdens of self-blame. The mind may quietly ask questions such as, "Why can't I do more?" or "Why am I struggling when others seem fine?" These thoughts often arise from comparing oneself to unrealistic expectations.

Self-blame can be particularly powerful when individuals feel that their limitations disrupt their goals or responsibilities. Moments of fatigue, cognitive difficulty, or emotional overwhelm may feel like personal failures rather than natural responses to neurological strain.

However, blaming oneself for the effects of a medical condition is both unfair and inaccurate. Hydrocephalus is not a reflection of character, discipline, or effort. It is a neurological reality that influences how the brain and body function. Recognizing this truth is an important step toward emotional freedom.

Letting go of self-blame does not mean abandoning responsibility for one's well-being. Instead, it means replacing guilt with understanding. It means acknowledging that the body and mind are doing their best within the circumstances they face.

When self-blame is released, emotional energy becomes available for healing. The mind begins to focus less on punishment and more on care, resilience, and forward movement.

Rewriting Inner Dialogue

Every person carries an internal voice that narrates their experiences. This voice can be encouraging and supportive, or it can be harsh and critical. Over time, repeated thoughts shape how individuals perceive themselves and their abilities.

For those living with hydrocephalus, the internal dialogue may sometimes become dominated by frustration or doubt. Thoughts such as "I should be doing better" or "I'm falling behind" may appear frequently, especially during moments of fatigue or stress.

Rewriting inner dialogue begins by noticing these thoughts without immediately accepting them as truth. The mind often repeats familiar patterns automatically, but awareness creates the opportunity to change those patterns.

A compassionate inner dialogue might replace harsh criticism with supportive language. Instead of thinking "I failed today," the mind might say, "Today was difficult, and I still showed up as best I could." This shift may seem small, but it changes the emotional tone of the entire experience.

Over time, practicing supportive self-talk can reshape how the brain processes challenges. Encouraging thoughts create emotional stability, helping individuals approach difficulties with patience rather than despair.

Honoring the Body's Limitations

The human body constantly communicates its needs through sensations such as fatigue, tension, and pain. For individuals living with hydrocephalus, these signals may appear more frequently due to neurological strain or cognitive effort.

Modern culture often promotes the idea that success requires pushing beyond limits at all costs. However, this mindset can be harmful for individuals whose bodies require careful pacing and recovery. Ignoring physical signals can increase exhaustion and emotional distress.

Honoring the body's limitations means listening to these signals with respect rather than frustration. Rest is not weakness. It is an essential form of maintenance for the brain and nervous system. Taking breaks, adjusting expectations, and pacing activities are ways of supporting long-term well-being.

When individuals learn to work with their bodies instead of against them, daily life becomes more sustainable. Energy can be used more effectively, and emotional stress decreases when expectations align with reality.

Honoring limitations also encourages self-trust. Instead of feeling betrayed by the body's needs, individuals begin to view those needs as valuable guidance for maintaining balance.

Celebrating Progress

Healing and personal growth often occur gradually, which can make progress difficult to recognize. When individuals focus only on large achievements, they may overlook the many small victories that happen along the way.

For someone living with hydrocephalus, progress might include completing a task despite fatigue, managing an anxious moment with breathing techniques, or reaching out for support during difficult times. These moments represent real strength and resilience.

Celebrating progress does not require grand ceremonies. Simple acknowledgments—such as writing down accomplishments, sharing successes with supportive people, or pausing to appreciate effort—can reinforce positive momentum.

Recognizing progress also shifts attention away from perceived shortcomings. Instead of focusing on what has not been achieved, the mind begins to see evidence of growth and capability.

Over time, these moments of recognition build confidence. They remind individuals that even small steps contribute to meaningful change.

Practicing Forgiveness Toward Oneself

Forgiveness is often associated with letting go of resentment toward others, but self-forgiveness can be equally powerful. Many people carry regrets, missed opportunities, or moments when they believe they did not handle situations perfectly.

Living with a neurological condition can intensify these feelings. Individuals may blame themselves for needing extra rest, canceling plans, or struggling to meet expectations. These thoughts can linger and create emotional weight.

Self-forgiveness involves recognizing that every person makes decisions based on the knowledge and energy available at the time. No one navigates life flawlessly. Mistakes, misjudgments, and setbacks are part of the human experience.

Letting go of self-directed resentment allows emotional wounds to heal. Forgiveness does not erase the past, but it frees individuals from repeatedly reliving moments of regret.

Through self-forgiveness, the mind learns to move forward with greater lightness and compassion.

Exercises

Exercise 1: The Compassionate Mirror

Step 1: Stand or sit in front of a mirror.

Step 2: Look at yourself gently without focusing on perceived flaws.

Step 3: Say three supportive statements to yourself aloud, such as "I am doing my best," or "My effort matters."

Step 4: Notice any emotions that arise while speaking these words.

Step 5: Repeat this practice regularly to strengthen self-kindness.

Exercise 2: Rewriting Self-Talk

Step 1: Write down a critical thought that frequently appears in your mind.

Step 2: Reflect on how this thought affects your emotions.

Step 3: Rewrite the thought using compassionate language.

Step 4: Read the new statement slowly and thoughtfully.

Step 5: Practice repeating the compassionate version whenever the original thought appears.

Exercise 3: The Progress Journal

Step 1: At the end of each day, write down three things you accomplished.

Step 2: Include small victories, such as resting when needed or completing a simple task.

Step 3: Reflect on the effort required to achieve each action.

Step 4: Express appreciation for your perseverance.

Step 5: Review your entries weekly to observe growth over time.

Journal Prompts

1. What forms of self-criticism appear most often in my thoughts?
2. How would I speak to a friend experiencing the same challenges?
3. What physical signals tell me that my body needs rest?
4. What small accomplishments have I overlooked recently?
5. How can I treat myself with greater patience during difficult days?
6. What past experiences do I need to forgive myself for?
7. What words of encouragement would support me today?
8. How can I celebrate progress without comparing myself to others?
9. What practices help me feel emotionally supported?
10. What does self-compassion mean to me personally?

Closing Reflection

Self-compassion is not weakness; it is a form of quiet strength. When individuals treat themselves with kindness, they create an internal environment where healing becomes possible.

Letting go of self-blame, honoring the body's needs, and celebrating progress all contribute to emotional restoration. Each act of self-forgiveness releases another layer of unnecessary burden.

The journey of healing is rarely perfect or predictable. Some days will bring clarity and confidence, while others may require patience and rest. Both experiences are natural parts of growth.

Through compassion and understanding, the inner landscape begins to soften. The mind becomes a place not of judgment, but of care—a space where resilience, healing, and hope can continue to grow.

Chapter 5: Creating a Mental Wellness Path

Understanding the Journey of Mental Wellness

Mental wellness is not a destination that is reached once and then permanently maintained. It is a path that unfolds day by day, shaped by choices, habits, and the way we respond to challenges. For individuals living with hydrocephalus, this path may involve unique obstacles such as neurological fatigue, fluctuating energy levels, and emotional stress connected to health concerns.

Rather than striving for constant emotional perfection, mental wellness involves building systems that support balance over time. It means creating daily rhythms that help the mind recover from stress, remain grounded during uncertainty, and maintain emotional resilience during difficult moments.

The concept of a "wellness path" recognizes that life naturally contains both calm and turbulence. Emotional waves, anxiety, and moments of discouragement are part of the human experience. What matters most is having supportive practices in place that guide the mind back toward stability.

Creating a wellness path also encourages individuals to think about mental health as an active process rather than something that simply happens. Small daily habits, such as reflection, rest, mindful breathing, and emotional awareness, gradually shape the mind's ability to adapt and recover.

Over time, these supportive practices become a foundation for resilience. They transform mental wellness from an abstract goal into a living routine that supports everyday life.

Building Sustainable Routines

Routines provide structure for the mind and body. When daily life contains predictable patterns, the nervous system experiences less uncertainty and stress. For individuals managing neurological conditions, routines can also help conserve energy and reduce cognitive strain.

A sustainable routine does not need to be rigid or overly complicated. In fact, overly strict schedules often create additional pressure. The most effective routines are flexible frameworks that support balance while allowing for rest when needed.

Morning rituals are often a helpful place to begin. Starting the day with a few calming practices—such as gentle stretching, quiet breathing, or reflective journaling—can create a sense of grounding before the day's responsibilities begin.

Evening routines can be equally valuable. Activities such as reducing screen time, reading quietly, or practicing relaxation exercises signal to the brain that it is time to slow down and recover. These routines help prepare the nervous system for restorative sleep.

Consistency is more important than intensity. Small daily practices repeated over time gradually strengthen emotional stability and mental clarity.

Mindful Reflection Practices

Reflection is a powerful tool for understanding emotional patterns and personal growth. Without moments of reflection, life can move so quickly that important insights are missed. Mindful reflection allows individuals to pause, observe their experiences, and learn from them.

Reflection can take many forms. Journaling is one of the most common methods, allowing thoughts and emotions to be expressed freely on paper. Writing often reveals patterns that may not be obvious during the busy flow of daily life.

Meditative reflection is another approach. Sitting quietly and observing thoughts without judgment allows the mind to process experiences in a calm environment. Over time, this practice strengthens awareness and reduces emotional reactivity.

Some individuals prefer creative forms of reflection such as drawing, music, or storytelling. These methods allow emotions to be expressed in ways that words alone may not capture.

Regular reflection builds emotional insight. It helps individuals recognize what supports their well-being and what creates unnecessary stress, allowing for thoughtful adjustments to daily habits.

Tracking Emotional Health

Just as physical health benefits from monitoring symptoms and progress, emotional health can also benefit from thoughtful observation. Tracking emotional experiences helps individuals identify patterns that might otherwise remain hidden.

For example, certain activities may consistently improve mood, while others may contribute to stress or exhaustion. Sleep quality, nutrition, social interactions, and environmental factors can all influence emotional well-being.

Tracking does not need to be complex. Some individuals use journals, calendars, or simple rating systems to record how they feel each day. Others prefer visual methods such as mood charts or color-coded systems that represent emotional states.

Over time, these records create a clearer picture of emotional patterns. Individuals may begin to notice that certain times of day, environments, or routines influence their mental state more strongly than expected.

This awareness provides valuable information for shaping healthier habits and creating supportive environments.

Strengthening Emotional Resilience

Resilience is the ability to recover from setbacks and continue moving forward despite difficulties. For individuals living with hydrocephalus, resilience often develops through repeated experiences of adaptation and perseverance.

Strengthening resilience begins with recognizing personal strengths. Many individuals underestimate their capacity to endure challenges, yet living with a neurological condition often requires remarkable courage and determination.

Resilience also grows through supportive relationships, self-compassion, and realistic expectations. When individuals accept that challenges are part of life rather than signs of failure, emotional recovery becomes easier.

Another key element of resilience is flexibility. The ability to adjust plans, expectations, and strategies allows individuals to navigate changing circumstances without becoming overwhelmed.

Resilience is not about ignoring difficulties or pretending everything is fine. Instead, it involves facing challenges with patience, creativity, and a willingness to continue growing.

Designing a Long-Term Wellness Plan

A long-term wellness plan is a personalized strategy for maintaining emotional balance over time. Rather than reacting to stress only after it becomes overwhelming, a wellness plan provides proactive guidance for supporting mental health.

This plan may include daily habits such as mindfulness practices, physical movement, social connection, and restful activities. It can also outline strategies for responding to difficult emotional periods when they arise.

One helpful approach is to think of the wellness plan as a flexible map rather than a strict rulebook. Life circumstances will change, and the plan should evolve accordingly.

Support systems are also an important part of long-term wellness. Friends, family members, healthcare providers, and community networks can provide encouragement and guidance when challenges arise.

When individuals create a thoughtful wellness plan, they develop a reliable framework for navigating life's emotional landscape with greater confidence and stability.

Exercises

Exercise 1: Designing Your Daily Wellness Routine

Step 1: Write down three small practices that help you feel calm or centered.

Step 2: Choose one practice to include in your morning routine.

Step 3: Choose another practice to include in your evening routine.

Step 4: Practice these routines consistently for one week.

Step 5: Reflect on how these routines affect your mood and energy levels.

Exercise 2: Emotional Pattern Mapping

Step 1: At the end of each day, rate your emotional state on a scale from 1 to 10.

Step 2: Write a short note about any events or activities that influenced your mood.

Step 3: Track sleep, physical energy, and stress levels alongside your emotional rating.

Step 4: Continue this practice for at least two weeks.

Step 5: Review your notes to identify patterns and insights about your emotional health.

Exercise 3: Personal Resilience Inventory

Step 1: Write down three challenges you have successfully navigated in the past.

Step 2: Reflect on the strengths or strategies that helped you overcome those challenges.

Step 3: Identify supportive people or resources that helped you during those times.

Step 4: Consider how these strengths can help you navigate current difficulties.

Step 5: Create a list of resilience reminders that you can revisit during challenging moments.

Journal Prompts

1. What daily habits support my emotional well-being?
2. When do I feel most mentally balanced?
3. What patterns have I noticed in my emotional health?
4. What activities restore my energy and focus?
5. How do supportive relationships influence my mental wellness?
6. What personal strengths help me face challenges?
7. What small changes could improve my daily routine?
8. How can I respond more compassionately to difficult days?
9. What would an ideal mental wellness routine look like for me?
10. What long-term goals do I have for emotional well-being?

Closing Reflection

Mental wellness is not created through one dramatic transformation but through many small acts of care repeated over time. Each moment of reflection, each calming breath, and each supportive routine strengthens the mind's capacity for balance.

By building sustainable habits, tracking emotional health, and developing a thoughtful wellness plan, individuals create a foundation that supports resilience and growth. These practices help transform uncertainty into opportunity for learning and self-understanding.

The path of mental wellness is deeply personal. It unfolds through patience, experimentation, and self-compassion. Some days will feel steady and clear, while others may require gentleness and rest.

What matters most is continuing to walk the path—step by step—knowing that each effort contributes to a stronger, more resilient mind.

Appendix A: 100 Mental Wellness Reflection Journal Prompts

Journaling is one of the most powerful tools for mental wellness. Writing creates a space where thoughts can slow down, emotions can be explored safely, and personal insight can develop over time. For individuals living with hydrocephalus or navigating mental health challenges, journaling provides a gentle method of listening to the mind without pressure or judgment.

The following prompts are designed to encourage reflection, emotional awareness, and personal growth. There are no right or wrong answers. Some prompts may resonate deeply, while others may simply spark curiosity. Write freely, honestly, and with compassion for yourself.

Take your time with these reflections. You may choose to explore one prompt per day, several prompts per week, or return to the same prompt multiple times as your perspective evolves.

Self-Awareness and Emotional Insight

1. What emotions have I been experiencing most frequently lately?
2. When do I feel the most emotionally balanced during the day?
3. What situations tend to create stress or anxiety for me?
4. What signs tell me that my mind needs rest?
5. How does my body communicate emotional tension?
6. What thoughts appear most often when I feel overwhelmed?
7. When do I feel the most mentally clear?
8. What activities help calm my mind?
9. What triggers emotional fatigue for me?
10. What does emotional balance feel like in my body?

Self-Compassion and Inner Dialogue

1. How do I speak to myself during difficult moments?
2. What would a compassionate inner voice sound like?
3. When was the last time I showed kindness toward myself?
4. What unrealistic expectations do I place on myself?
5. How can I respond more gently to my mistakes?
6. What does self-compassion mean to me?
7. How would I support a friend facing my current challenges?
8. What words of encouragement do I need to hear right now?
9. How can I practice patience with myself today?
10. What strengths do I often overlook in myself?

Anxiety and Emotional Regulation

1. What situations tend to trigger my anxiety?
2. What physical sensations appear when I feel anxious?
3. What thoughts accompany my anxious moments?
4. What grounding techniques help me regain calm?
5. What environments make me feel safe and relaxed?
6. How can I prepare for stressful situations in advance?
7. What small habits help reduce anxiety in my daily life?
8. What reassurances can I offer myself during worry?
9. When has anxiety taught me something valuable?
10. How can I support my nervous system during stressful days?

Depression and Emotional Recovery

1. What signs indicate that I may be entering a depressive cycle?
2. What small actions help me regain motivation?
3. What activities once brought me joy?
4. How can I gently reintroduce those activities into my life?
5. What thoughts appear during moments of emotional heaviness?
6. What sources of hope exist in my life right now?
7. What supportive people or communities help me feel less alone?
8. How can I show myself compassion during difficult days?
9. What does healing look like for me right now?
10. What reminds me that emotional darkness is temporary?

Mindfulness and Presence

1. What helps me stay present in the moment?
2. How does my breathing change when I am calm?
3. What sensory experiences bring me peace?
4. How does nature influence my emotional state?
5. What thoughts arise when I sit quietly with myself?
6. What moments today made me feel grounded?
7. How can I bring more mindful awareness into daily activities?
8. What distractions pull me away from the present moment?
9. How can I gently guide my attention back to the present?
10. What does stillness feel like in my mind?

Personal Growth and Resilience

1. What challenges have I overcome in the past?
2. What strengths helped me through those experiences?
3. How has living with hydrocephalus shaped my resilience?
4. What lessons have emerged from difficult times?
5. What personal qualities am I developing through adversity?
6. What does resilience mean in my life?
7. How do I adapt when plans change unexpectedly?
8. What encourages me to keep moving forward?
9. What personal growth am I experiencing right now?
10. How can I honor my progress?

Relationships and Support

1. Who are the people who support my well-being?
2. How can I strengthen those connections?
3. What does healthy communication look like for me?
4. How do I express my needs to others?
5. What boundaries help protect my emotional health?
6. How can I ask for support when I need it?
7. What relationships bring me the most comfort?
8. What relationships create emotional strain?
9. How can I nurture mutual understanding with others?
10. What does emotional safety feel like in relationships?

Daily Habits and Wellness

1. What daily habits support my mental health?
2. What routines help stabilize my mood?
3. How does sleep affect my emotional well-being?
4. What physical activities help restore my energy?
5. How does nutrition influence my mental clarity?
6. What calming rituals can I add to my day?
7. How do breaks and rest improve my focus?
8. What habits contribute to emotional stress?
9. What small changes could improve my daily routine?
10. What does a balanced day look like for me?

Hope, Purpose, and Future Vision

1. What gives my life meaning?
2. What dreams still inspire me?
3. How can I nurture hope during difficult times?
4. What future experiences would I like to explore?
5. How can I align my daily actions with my values?
6. What brings me a sense of purpose?
7. What does emotional healing look like in the future?
8. What qualities do I want to cultivate in myself?
9. How can I continue growing despite challenges?
10. What possibilities exist beyond my current struggles?

Gratitude and Positive Reflection

1. What am I grateful for today?
2. What small moments brought me peace recently?
3. What positive changes have I noticed in my life?
4. Who has shown kindness toward me lately?
5. What personal accomplishments deserve recognition?
6. What beauty did I notice in the world today?
7. What strengths helped me navigate this week?
8. What makes life meaningful even during difficulty?
9. What brings warmth or comfort to my heart?
10. What message of encouragement would I give my future self?

Closing Reflection

Reflection is a powerful act of self-care. Each time you pause to write, you create a quiet space where your thoughts and emotions can be understood rather than rushed or ignored. Over time, journaling becomes more than a simple activity—it becomes a dialogue with your inner self.

These prompts are not meant to be completed perfectly or quickly. Some may open doors to deeper understanding, while others may simply provide a moment of calm reflection. What matters most is the willingness to listen to your own thoughts with patience and curiosity.

Living with hydrocephalus or navigating mental health challenges can sometimes feel overwhelming, but reflection reminds us that growth often occurs in small, quiet moments of awareness. Each page written is a step toward greater understanding, resilience, and emotional balance.

As you continue your journaling journey, remember that healing does not require perfection. It grows through honesty, self-compassion, and the courage to explore your own inner landscape. Within those reflections lies the potential for clarity, strength, and renewal.

Message from the Author:

I hope you enjoyed this book, I love astrology and knew there was not a book such as this out on the shelf. I love metaphysical items as well. Please check out my other books:

-Life of Government Benefits

-My life of Hell

-My life with Hydrocephalus

-Red Sky

-World Domination:Woman's rule

-World Domination:Woman's Rule 2: The War

-Life and Banishment of Apophis: book 1

-The Kidney Friendly Diet

-The Ultimate Hemp Cookbook

-Creating a Dispensary(legally)

-Cleanliness throughout life: the importance of showering from childhood to adulthood.

-Strong Roots: The Risks of Overcoddling children

-Hemp Horoscopes: Cosmic Insights and Earthly Healing

- Celestial Hemp Navigating the Zodiac: Through the Green Cosmos

-Astrological Hemp: Aligning The Stars with Earth's Ancient Herb

-The Astrological Guide to Hemp: Stars, Signs, and Sacred Leaves

-Green Growth: Innovative Marketing Strategies for your Hemp Products and Dispensary

-Cosmic Cannabis

-Astrological Munchies

-Henry The Hemp

-Zodiacal Roots: The Astrological Soul Of Hemp

- **Green Constellations: Intersection of Hemp and Zodiac**

-Hemp in The Houses: An astrological Adventure Through The Cannabis Galaxy

-Galactic Ganja Guide

Heavenly Hemp
Zodiac Leaves
Doctor Who Astrology
Cannastrology
Stellar Satvias and Cosmic Indicas
Celestial Cannabis: A Zodiac Journey
AstroHerbology: The Sky and The Soil: Volume 1
AstroHerbology:Celestial Cannabis:Volume 2
Cosmic Cannabis Cultivation
The Starry Guide to Herbal Harmony: Volume 1
The Starry Guide to Herbal Harmony: Cannabis Universe: Volume 2
Yugioh Astrology: Astrological Guide to Deck, Duels and more
Nightmare Mansion: Echoes of The Abyss
Nightmare Mansion 2: Legacy of Shadows
Nightmare Mansion 3: Shadows of the Forgotten
Nightmare Mansion 4: Echoes of the Damned
The Life and Banishment of Apophis: Book 2
Nightmare Mansion: Halls of Despair
Healing with Herb: Cannabis and Hydrocephalus
Planetary Pot: Aligning with Astrological Herbs: Volume 1
Fast Track to Freedom: 30 Days to Financial Independence Using AI, Assets, and Agile Hustles
Cosmic Hemp Pathways
How to Become Financially Free in 30 Days: 10,000 Paths to Prosperity
Zodiacal Herbage: Astrological Insights: Volume 1
Nightmare Mansion: Whispers in the Walls
The Daleks Invade Atlantis
Henry the hemp and Hydrocephalus

10X The Kidney Friendly Diet
Cannabis Universe: Adult coloring book

Hemp Astrology: The Healing Power of the Stars

Zodiacal Herbage: Astrological Insights: Cannabis Universe: Volume 2

Planetary Pot: Aligning with Astrological Herbs: Cannabis Universes: Volume 2

Doctor Who: Convergence Protocol – The Replicator War

Nightmare Mansion: Curse of the Blood Moon

The Celestial Stoner: A Guide to the Zodiac

Cosmic Pleasures: Sex Toy Astrology for Every Sign

Hydrocephalus Astrology: Navigating the Stars and Healing Waters

Lapis and the Mischievous Chocolate Bar

Celestial Positions: Sexual Astrology for Every Sign

Apophis's Shadow Work Journal: : A Journey of Self-Discovery and Healing

Kinky Cosmos: Sexual Kink Astrology for Every Sign

Digital Cosmos: The Astrological Digimon Compendium

Stellar Seeds: The Cosmic Guide to Growing with Astrology

Apophis's Daily Gratitude Journal

Cat Astrology: Feline Mysteries of the Cosmos

The Cosmic Kama Sutra: An Astrological Guide to Sexual Positions

Unleash Your Potential: A Guided Journal Powered by AI Insights

Whispers of the Enchanted Grove

Cosmic Pleasures: An Astrological Guide to Sexual Kinks

369, 12 Manifestation Journal

Whisper of the nocturne journal(blank journal for writing or drawing)

The Boogey Book

Locked In Reflection: A Chastity Journey Through Locktober

Generating Wealth Quickly:How to Generate $100,000 in 24 Hours

Star Magic: Harness the Power of the Universe

The Flatulence Chronicles: A Fart Journal for Self-Discovery

The Doctor and The Death Moth

Seize the Day: A Personal Seizure Tracking Journal

The Ultimate Boogeyman Safari: A Journey into the Boogie World and Beyond

Whispers of Samhain: 1,000 Spells of Love, Luck, and Lunar Magic: Samhain Spell Book

Apophis's guides:Witch's Spellbook Crafting Guide for Halloween

Frost & Flame: The Enchanted Yule Grimoire of 1000 Winter Spells

The Ultimate Boogey Goo Guide & Spooky Activities for Halloween Fun

Harmony of the Scales: A Libra's Spellcraft for Balance and Beauty

The Enchanted Advent: 36 Days of Christmas Wonders

Nightmare Mansion: The Labyrinth of Screams

Harvest of Enchantment: 1,000 Spells of Gratitude, Love, and Fortune for Thanksgiving

The Boogey Chronicles: A Journal of Nightly Encounters and Shadowy Secrets

The 12 Days of Financial Freedom: A Step-by-Step Christmas Countdown to Transform Your Finances

Sigil of the Eternal Spiral Blank Journal

A Christmas Feast: Timeless Recipes for Every Meal

Holiday Stress-Free Solutions: A Survival Guide to Thriving During the Festive Season

Yu-Gi-Oh! Holiday Gifting Mastery: The Ultimate Guide for Fans and Newcomers Alike

Holiday Harmony: A Hydrocephalus Survival Guide for the Festive Season

Celestial Craft: The Witch's Almanac for 2025 – A Cosmic Guide to Manifestations, Moons, and Mystical Events

Doctor Who: The Toymaker's Winter Wonderland

Tulsa King Unveiled: A Thrilling Guide to Stallone's Mafia Masterpiece

Pendulum Craft: A Complete Guide to Crafting and Using Personalized Divination Tools

Nightmare Mansion: Santa's Eternal Eve

Starlight Noel: A Cosmic Journey through Christmas Mysteries

The Dark Architect: Unlocking the Blueprint of Existence

Surviving the Embrace: The Ultimate Guide to Encounters with The Hugging Molly

The Enchanted Codex: Secrets of the Craft for Witches, Wiccans, and Pagans

Harvest of Gratitude: A Complete Thanksgiving Guide

Yuletide Essentials: A Complete Guide to an Authentic and Magical Christmas

Celestial Smokes: A Cosmic Guide to Cigars and Astrology

Living in Balance: A Comprehensive Survival Guide to Thriving with Diabetes Insipidus

Cosmic Symbiosis: The Venom Zodiac Chronicles

The Cursed Paw of Ambition

Cosmic Symbiosis: The Astrological Venom Journal

Celestial Wonders Unfold: A Stargazer's Guide to the Cosmos (2024-2029)

The Ultimate Black Friday Prepper's Guide: Mastering Shopping Strategies and Savings

Cosmic Sales: The Astrological Guide to Black Friday Shopping

Legends of the Corn Mother and Other Harvest Myths

Whispers of the Harvest: The Corn Mother's Journal

The Evergreen Spellbook

The Doctor Meets the Boogeyman

The White Witch of Rose Hall's SpellBook

The Gingerbread Golem's Shadow: A Study in Sweet Darkness

The Gingerbread Golem Codex: An Academic Exploration of Sweet Myths

The Gingerbread Golem Grimoire: Sweet Magicks and Spells for the Festive Witch

The Curse of the Gingerbread Golem

10-minute Christmas Crafts for kids

Christmas Crisis Solutions: The Ultimate Last-Minute Survival Guide

Gingerbread Golem Recipes: Holiday Treats with a Magical Twist

The Infinite Key: Unlocking Mystical Secrets of the Ages

Enchanted Yule: A Wiccan and Pagan Guide to a Magical and Memorable Season

Dinosaurs of Power: Unlocking Ancient Magick

Astro-Dinos: The Cosmic Guide to Prehistoric Wisdom

Gallifrey's Yule Logs: A Festive Doctor Who Cookbook

The Dino Grimoire: Secrets of Prehistoric Magick

The Gift They Never Knew They Needed

The Gingerbread Golem's Culinary Alchemy: Enchanting Recipes for a Sweetly Dark Feast

A Time Lord Christmas: Holiday Adventures with the Doctor

Krampusproofing Your Home: Defensive Strategies for Yule

Silent Frights: A Collection of Christmas Creepypastas to Chill Your Bones

Santa Raptor's Jolly Carnage: A Dino-Claus Christmas Tale

Prehistoric Palettes: A Dino Wicca Coloring Journey

The Christmas Wishkeeper Chronicles

The Starlight Sleigh: A Holiday Journey

Elf Secrets: The True Magic of the North Pole

Candy Cane Conjurations

Cooking with Kids: Recipes Under 20 Minutes

Doctor Who: The TARDIS Confiscation

The Anxiety First Aid Kit: Quick Tools to Calm Your Mind

Frosty Whispers: A Winter's Tale

The Infinite Key: Unlocking the Secrets to Prosperity, Resilience, and Purpose

The Grasping Void: Why You'll Regret This Purchase

Astrology for Busy Bees: Star Signs Simplified

The Instant Focus Formula: Cut Through the Noise

The Secret Language of Colors: Unlocking the Emotional Codes

Sacred Fossil Chronicles: Blank Journal

The Christmas Cottage Miracle

Feeding Frenzy: Graboid-Inspired Recipes

Manifest in Minutes: The Quick Law of Attraction Guide

The Symbiote Chronicles: Doctor Who's Venomous Journey

Think Tiny, Grow Big: The Minimalist Mindset

The Energy Key: Unlocking Limitless Motivation

New Year, New Magic: Manifesting Your Best Year Yet

Unstoppable You: Mastering Confidence in Minutes

Infinite Energy: The Secret to Never Feeling Drained

Lightning Focus: Mastering the Art of Productivity in a Distracted World

Saturnalia Manifestation Magick: A Guide to Unlocking Abundance During the Solstice

Graboids and Garland: The Ultimate Tremors-Themed Christmas Guide

12 Nights of Holiday Magic

The Power of Pause: 60-Second Mindfulness Practices

The Quick Reset: How to Reclaim Your Life After Burnout

The Shadow Eater: A Tale of Despair and Survival

The Micro-Mastery Method: Transform Your Skills in Just Minutes a Day

Reclaiming Time: How to Live More by Doing Less

Chronovore: The Eternal Nexus

The Mind Reset: Unlocking Your Inner Peace in a Chaotic World
Confidence Code: Building Unshakable Self-Belief
Baby the Vampire Terrier
Baby the Vampire Terrier's Christmas Adventure
Celestial Streams: The Content Creator's Astrology Manual
The Wealth Whisperer: Unlocking Abundance with Everyday Actions
The Energy Equation: Maximize Your Output Without Burning Out
The Happiness Algorithm: Science-Backed Steps to Joyful Living
Stress-Free Success: Achieving Goals Without Anxiety
Mindful Wealth: The New Blueprint for Financial Freedom
The Festive Flavors of New Year: A Culinary Celebration
The Master's Gambit: Keys of Eternal Power
Shadowed Secrets: Groundhog Day Mysteries
Beneath the Burrow: Lessons from the Groundhog
Spring's Whispers: The Groundhog's Prediction
The Limitless Mindset: Unlock Your Untapped Potential
The Focus Funnel: How to Cut Through Chaos and Get Results
Bold Moves: Building Courage to Live on Your Terms
The Daily Shift: Simple Practices for Lasting Transformation
The Quarter-Life Reset: Thriving in Your 20s and 30s
The Art of Shadowplay: Building Your Own Personal Myth
The Eternal Loop: Finding Purpose in Repetition
Burrowing Wisdom: Life Lessons from the Groundhog
Shadow Work: A Groundhog Day Perspective
Love in Bloom: 5-Minute Romantic Gestures
The Shadowspell Codex: Secrets of Forbidden Magick
The Burnout Cure: Finding Balance in a Busy World
The Groundhog Prophecy: Unlocking Seasonal Secrets
Nog Tales: The Spirited History of Eggnog
Six More Weeks: Embracing Seasonal Transitions
The Lumivian Chronicles: Fragments of the Fifth Dimension

Money on Your Mind: A Beginner's Guide to Wealth
The Focus Fix: Breaking Through Distraction
January's Spirit Keepers: Mystical Protectors of the Cold
Creativity Unchained: Unlocking Your Wildest Ideas in 2025
Manifestation Mastery: 365 Days to Rewrite Your Reality
The Groundhog's Mirror: Reflecting on Change
The Weeping Angels' Christmas Curse
Burrowed in Time: A Groundhog Day Journey
Heartbeats: Poems to Share with Your Valentine
Dino Wicca: The Sacred Grimoire of Prehistoric Magick
Courage of the Pride: Finding Your Inner Roar
The Lion's Leap: Bold Moves for Big Results
Healthy Hustle: Achieving Without Overworking
Practical Manifesting: Turning Dreams into Reality in 2025
Jurassic Pharaohs: Unlocking the Magick of Ancient Egypt and Dino Wicca
The Happiness Equation: Small Changes for Big Joy
The Confidence Compass: Finding Your Inner Strength
Whispers in the Hollow: Tales of the Forgotten Beasts
Echoes from the Hollow: The Return of Forgotten Beasts
The Hollow Ascendant: The Rise of the Forgotten Beasts
The Relationship Reset: Building Better Connections
Mastering the Morning: How to Win the Day Before 8 AM
The Shadow's Dance: Groundhog Day Symbolism
Cupid's Kitchen: Quick Valentine's Day Recipes
Valentine's Day on a Budget: Love Without Breaking the Bank
Astrocraft: Aligning the Stars in the World of Minecraft
Forecasting Life: Groundhog Day Reflections

Bleeding Hearts: Twisted Tales of Valentine's Terror

Herbal Smoke Revolution: The Ultimate Guide to Nature's Cigarette Alternative

Winter's Wrath: The Complete Survival Blueprint for Extreme Freezes.

The Groundhog's Shadow: A Tale of Seasons
Burrowed Insights: Wisdom from the Groundhog
Sensual Strings: The Art of Erotic Bondage
Whispered Flames: Unlocking the Power of Fire Play
Forgotten Shadows: A Guide to Cryptids Lost to Time
Six Weeks of Secrets: Groundhog Day's Hidden Messages
Shadows and Cycles: Groundhog Day Reflections
The Art of Love Letters: Crafting the Perfect Message
Romantic Getaways at Home: Turning Your Space into Paradise
Purrfect Brews: A Cat Lover's Guide to Coffee and Companionship
The Groundhog's Wisdom: Timeless Lessons for Modern Life
The Shadow Oracle: Groundhog Day as a Predictor
Emerging from the Burrow: A Journey of Renewal
The Language of Love: Learning Your Partner's Love Style
Authorpreneur: The Ultimate Blueprint for Writing, Publishing, and Thriving as an Author
Weathering the Seasons: Groundhog Day Perspectives
Valentine's Day Magic: A Guide to Romantic Rituals
The Shadow Chronicles: Stories of Groundhog Day
Love and Laughter: Fun Games for Valentine's Day
AstroRealty: Unlocking the Stars for Property Success
The Groundhog's Path: A Guide to Seasonal Balance
Groundhog Day Diaries: Reflections in the Shadow
The Groundhog's Light: Illuminating the Path Ahead
Valentine's Traditions from Around the World
AI Wealth Revolution: Unlocking the Trillionaire Mindset
Love Rekindled: Reigniting Passion in Relationships
Single and Thriving: Self-Love on Valentine's Day
Emerald Legends: Mystical Tales of Ireland
Green Alchemy: Harnessing Nature's Magic
The Hearts of Horror: A Valentine's Day Nightmare

The Leprechaun's Guide to Wealth and Wisdom

Dancing with the Sidhe: Celebrating the Otherworld

Shamrocks and Shadows: Mysteries of the Green Isle

Emerald Energy: Harnessing Luck and Growth

The Gingerbread Golem's Valentine: A Sweetheart's Guide to Love and Enchantment

The Celtic Knot: Weaving Life and Destiny

Green Fire: Elemental Magic for St. Patrick's Day

Clover Chronicles: Finding Your Inner Luck

Ireland's Mystical Creatures: A Field Guide

Gingerbread Golem's Love Almanac

Prowl and Thrive: The Lion's Guide to Success

Love Alchemy: Transforming Your Life Through Heart Energy

WORLD DOMINATION: Woman's Rule 3:The New Life

The Midnight Rose: A Guide to Lunar Love Spells

The Forbidden Letters: Writing Your Own Love Prophecy

Luck and Lore: St. Patrick's Day for Modern Mystics

The Green Path: A Pagan Celebration of Renewal

The Dark Architect's Guide to Reprogramming Reality

Prankster's Paradise: A Guide to Harmless Hijinks

Manifest Your Reality: The Law of Attraction Simplified

The TARDIS Owner's Manual: Understanding the Doctor's Ship: *A complete guide to the TARDIS, its technology, secrets, and mysteries*

Starlit Romance: Astrology Secrets for Finding True Love

The Time Lord's Atlas: A Complete Guide to the Whoniverse: ***A breakdown of the locations, planets, and dimensions explored in Doctor Who***

Sweetheart Shadows: The Dark Side of Love and Attraction

February Fire: Reigniting Passion in Every Area of Life

The Self-Love Toolkit: 5 Ways to Embrace Who You Are

February Sparks: Ignite Your Dreams in 28 Days

March to Success: A 31-Day Action Blueprint
Ancient Paths: The 13 Sacred Principles of Dino Wicca
Echoes of Tomorrow: Navigating the AI Revolution
The Wellness Blueprint: Balancing Mind, Body, and Soul
Green Horizons: Sustainable Living for a Better Tomorrow
The AI Wealth Code: How to Make Millions with Automation
AI-Powered Creativity: Writing, Art, and Music for Profit
Extinction Rites: Rebirthing Your Soul Through Prehistoric Magick
Sacred Serpents tarot
Celestial Enchantment blank journal
Star Strains
Culinary Journeys: Exploring Global Flavors at Home
The Hollowvale Curse
The Hollowvale Harvest
The Egg of Transformation: Awakening Your Inner Power
Blooming Into Power: A Wiccan Guide to Spring Awakening
The Nightmare Nexus: The Third Doctor's Perilous Haunting
Digital Detox: Reclaiming Your Life in a Connected World
Ostara's Path: Walking the Spiral of Renewal
The Sacred Hare
Financial Freedom: Building Wealth in the Modern Age
Spring's Cauldron: Stirring the Waters of Change
The Hollowvale Pact
Quantum Consciousness: The Science of Reality Shifting
The Hollowvale Hunger
The Sacred Waters Within: A Witch's Guide to Hydrocephalus Magick
The Raven's Nest: Building a Life of Unshakable Stability
AI and the Human Mind: The Future of Intelligence
The Hollowvale Reckoning
Timeless Love: Building and Maintaining Lasting Relationships

The Raven's Roar: Unlocking Unstoppable Confidence
Raven Sight: Awakening Intuition and Inner Wisdom
The Butterfly Effect: Small Changes, Big Transformations
Taming the Boogeyman: How to Conquer Your Inner Fears
The Magick of Green: Awakening Earth's Energy in You
The Entrepreneurial Mindset: Secrets to Business Success
The Hollowvale End
The Shadow Luck Ritual: Reclaiming Power from Your Dark Side
Spring Magick for Beginners: A Simple Guide to Seasonal Energy Work
Doctor Who: The Hollowvale Conundrum
The March of Miracles: Unlocking Synchronicities in Spring
Unveiling the Cosmos: A Guide to Stargazing and Space Exploration
The Ultimate Guide to Surviving an Economic Collapse
The AI Gold Rush: How to Profit from the AI Revolution
Bastet's Shadow: The Hidden Power of Feline Magick
The Bastet Codex: Unlocking the Goddess's Magickal Secrets
Purring Spells: Harnessing Bastet's Healing Frequencies
Bastet's Nine Lives: Rebirth, Transformation, and Immortality Spells
Primal Currents: Hydrocephalus Magick in the Path of Dino Wicca
The Digital Gold Rush: Mastering E-Commerce and Online Sales
Future Shock: Adapting to the Next Decade of Change
The Quantum Mindset: Think Like a Billionaire
Sacred Motherhood: Awakening the Divine Feminine Within
The Mother's Spellbook: Enchantments for Love, Protection, and Prosperity
The Witch's Guide to Parenting: Raising Empowered and Intuitive Children

The Magick of Motherhood: Reclaiming Your Power Through Rituals

The Pagan Path to Self-Love: A Goddess's Guide to Worth and Confidence

Wild Woman Magick: Unleashing Your Primal Power

The Money Magnet Blueprint: Unlocking Unlimited Wealth

Biohacking 101: Unlock Your Body's Full Potential

The Wild Father: A Pagan Guide to Strength and Wisdom

The Sacred Masculine: Unlocking Your Inner Power

The Druid's Compass

The Warrior's Mindset

The Father's Fire

Odin's Path

Ancestral Bonds

The House That Whispers

The Magician's Code

The Wild Hunt

The Green Man's Path

The Altar of Success

The Shadow and the Sword

The High Priestess's Guide to Energy Healing

The Lunar Mother

The Sacred Self-Care Grimoire

The Womb Wisdom Codex

The Wheel of the Mother

The Witch's Guide to Manifestation

The Q2 Reset

The Ultimate Guide to AI-Powered Passive Income

Escape the 9-5

AI Feline Fortunes

The Tear-Stained Grimoire

Razorblade Runes

Cemetery Sirens

The Midnight Wristwatch
The Town That Forgets
AI Horror & Creepypasta
The Hollow Frequency
The Breach Echo
The Quiet Between Worlds
The Sigil of Tharan-Khul
Summon the Vault of Y'ha'ten
The Becoming Codex
The Profit of Az'ra-nar
The Drowned Logos
Echoes of the Eldritch Will
The Deep Ledger
Necronomicon of Networth
Covenant of the Wealthwyrm
The Whisperer's Manifesto
The Rites of Azh-K'luth
The Ark of the Crawling Coin
The Tithe of Shadows
Inkheart Abyss
The Timewinds of Y'ha-nthlei
The Spiral Labyrinth of Azag-Nirrh
The Gallifreyan Heresy of the Black Pharaoh
The Psalms of Nyog-Sotha
Black Rain Alchemy
The Infinite Maw
The Entropic Blueprint
The Oracle of Sh'guul
The Book of Breach
The Drowned Saint's Testament
Dreamcraft of the Sleeper God
The Silence Market
Cthonomics: The Dark Wealth Algorithm

Invocation of the Ten-Eyed King
Wealthbound to the Wyrm Below
Become the Unnameable
Codex of the Sovereign Flame
Rituals of Relentless Becoming
The Shadow Ascends
The Eyes Beneath You
The Will That Wakes Worlds
Silence Is a Weapon
The Mirror That Screams
The Whisper Between Moments
The Mind That Devours Fear
The Myth of the Finished Self
The Architect of Your Madness
The Voice You've Buried
The Discipline of Madness
Stormborn: Awakening Your Inner Tempest
The Mind That Ate Time
Unbind Your Becoming
The Pact You Owe Yourself
The Devourer's Diet
The Acid That Carves the Path
The Tower You Must Burn
The Breath Between Worlds
Speak Like the Deep
The Labyrinth Within
The Spine of the Sea God
Rejection Is a Portal
The Crown You Refused
The Scar Is the Spell
The Lightless Flame
The Habit of Becoming Horrific
ChickenJockey Chaos

The Gatekeeper Within
You Are Not Your Name
The Compass of the Mad
The Archive of Unsent Letters
What the Mirror Can't Show You
The Knife You Needed
Worship Nothing, Become Everything
The Other Voice
The Body the World Forgot
The Vein of the Void
The Black Bone Codex
The Puzzle of the Hidden Self (Millennium Puzzle)
The Eye That Sees the Lie *(Millennium Eye)*
The Ring of Return (Millennium Ring)
The Rod of Relentless Will ***(Millennium Rod)***
The Tally of the Soul (Millennium Tauk/Necklace)
The Key to the Locked Timeline (Millennium Key)
The Scale of Sacred Decisions (Millennium Scales)
Inferno Bites: The UnOfficial Minecraft Lava Cookbook
Rot in the Attic
Prana: The Hidden Force of Your Infinite Self
The Shadow Realm Within: Transforming Darkness Into Destiny
The Borderland Collapse
Claws of Protection: Bastet's Defensive Magick
Mr. Ring-a-Ding's Madness
Yugioh Astrology: Celestial Deckcraft and Duel Destiny (2026–2027 Edition)
The Seal You Signed: Unlocking the Power You Once Feared
The Puzzle of Infinite Minds: Unlocking the Mentalism Hidden Within
The Eye That Mirrors the All: Secrets of Inner Reflection
Doctor Who: The Toymaker's Broadcast

The Rod of Eternal Flow: Commanding the Currents of Vibration
Golden Eyes of Bastet: Enhancing Psychic Vision
The Key of Dual Forces: Balance Within the Polarity
The Scales of Living Rhythm: Timing the Dance of Life
The Necklace of Hidden Cause: Weaving the Webs of Fate
The Ring of Secret Masters: Rising Through the All Within All
Daggers of the Dying Deep
Bastet's Wealth and Fortune Magick: Prosperity Rituals of the Goddess
The Tide that Speaks
The Scrolls of Petosiris: 13 Rituals from the Feathered Eye
Petosiris and the Living Plague of Osirion
Feline Fire: Bastet's Passion and Love Magick
The Star Altar of Petosiris
Bastet's Whiskers: Supernatural Sensory Magick
The Bastet Grimoire
Feeding the Shadows
The Mouthless Prayer
The Spiral Wound
Becoming the Ibis: Lessons from Petosiris's Mind
The Crimson Coven: Cola Magick for Sweet Dominion
Sacred Cat's Paw
The Soda Zodiac: A Flavor for Every Sign
Covenant of the Crawling Flame
The Ink of Ish'Zur
Frothroot: The Thirst That Ate the World
The Golden Glyphs of Prosperity
The Etherbind Codex
Echoes of the Resistance: Reclaiming the You That Survived
Harnessed Minds: Breaking Free from Mental Control
The Eyes in the Smoke

Rootwake: The Carbon Covenant
Skitter Logic: Unlearning the Fear That Built You
Doctor Who: The World That Froths
Rootwake: The Fizz That Rewrites Flesh
Rootwake: Frothfather of the World
The Holly Pact: Blood Beneath the Mistletoe
The 2nd Mass Principle: Building Unbreakable Tribes
Web of Wits: A Survival Guide to Encounters with Anasi the Spider (Aunt Nancy)
The Hexbreaking Handbook: Effective Spells to Remove Curses
Pop Alchemy: Transform Your Life One Sip at a Time
The Mason Code: Leading in Unleadable Times
Petosiris and the Fifth Chamber of Thoth
The Ether Seed Within
The Parent of Tomorrow
Petosiris's Pyramid of Perpetual Wealth
Unlearn the World
Grimoire of the Hollow Tongue
Zodiac Weeds: Finding Your Strain Through the Stars
Aquarius Rises in the Bank
The Sugar God's Smile
The Skinclock Reversal: Biohacking the Face of Time
Debtburn: How to Obliterate What You Owe Forever
The Ice Cream Oracle: What Your Cone Says About Your Future
Silence Is Sovereignty: The Power of Being Unreadable
The Wind That Whispers Through Stone
Path of the Four Directions
Doctor Who: The Maestro's Symphony of Endings
Oxygen Grail: Breathing to Undo the Clock
Zodiacal Collapse: When Stars Devour Time
Teachings from the Red Sand Silence

Doctor Who: Omega – The Broken Equation
Memory Wipe Your Past: Start Over Like a MiB
Mitochondria Prime: Ignite the Core of Youth
A Nest of Roaches
Grub from the Galaxy: MiB Recipes You'll Never Forget
Whiskers of Power: Bastet's Guide to Inner Sovereignty
The Gift Must Cost Them: Negotiation Through Unequal Exchange
The Worm Guys' Wealth Code: Hustle Like an Alien
Bug Out: The Edgar Method for Ruthless Goal Setting
Weaving Life with Spiderwoman's Pattern
Doctor Who: The Rani's Renaissance
How to Get a Job (If You're a Puppygirl)
Speak Through Others: The Art of Proxy Power
T-Rex Your Trauma: Reclaim the Power of Your Primal Self
The Black Briefcase: How MiB Stay Wealthy in Silence
The Thirst Beyond Reason: Understanding Diabetes Insipidus From the Inside Out
Backwoods Witchcraft for Billionaires: The Pagan Path from Dirt Roads to Gold Roads
The Moonshine Grimoire: Fermented Spells for Abundance
The Nameless Geometry
The Wraith's Mixtape: Spellcasting with Songs of Sorrow
The Gallifreyan Gentleman: Silent Wealth, Sonic Confidence, and the Doctor's Code of Living
Sugar Water Confidence
Dino Totems: Spirit Guides from Earth's First Gods
Pumpkin Sigils & Ritual Smoke
The Hózhó Compass
The Distortus Discipline – Order from Inner Mutation
Witchcraft for the Cold-Blooded Soul
Moonlight Over the Blessingway
Water, Interrupted: When the Body Forgets How to Hold On

Deformed but Divine: Embracing Your Asymmetry
Hexes in the Henhouse: The Farm Witch's Guide to Power
The Reversed Flame: A Grimoire of Inverted Power
Salt, Cells, and Sanity: Reclaiming Balance with Diabetes Insipidus
King of the Broken: Crowning the Flawed Self
Moonlight Scars: Emo Moon Magick and the Art of Lunar Sorrow
Noose Spells: Magick of the Hanging Rope
The Goth Cathedral: Rituals of the Broken and Beautiful
The Cretaceous Codex: Dino Spirits and Fossil Magick
The Turkey Bones Ritual
Nine Lives of Manifestation: Unlocking Bastet's Reality Codes
Chaos Muscles: Building Strength from Twisted Pain
Emo Blood Magick: The Veins of Power
The 3AM Flood: Nighttime Urination, Sleep Loss, and the DI Spiral
The Silence Between the Stars
The Lemon Method: Sour Your Way to Success
Starlit Sovereign
The Rite of Twelve Gates: Walking the Gates of the Duat.
Cornbread and Conjure: Recipes for Riches and Rootwork
The Black Rose Rituals: Emo Love Spells and Obsession Magick
The Eternal Goodbye: Death Magick and Rebirth Rituals
Sinkrot: The Drain That Remembers
The Hybrid Mindset: Thinking Beyond Evolution
Bone Dry: Navigating Dehydration Before It Breaks You
Wreathcraft: Winter Sigils and Yuletide Spells
The Rite of Twelve Mouths
S'mores of the Damned: Haunted Recipes for Halloween Night

Rethink the Drink: A Beverage Survival Guide for DI Warriors

The Shadow Chord: Guitar Magick and Sonic

Malformed Yet Majestic: Leading When You Feel Wrong Inside

The Cursed Diary: Ink-Stained Spells of the Emo Soul

Anxiety Off Switch: Emergency Reset for a Fried Nervous System

The Energy Heist: How to Take Back Your Life from Drainers

Beyond the Bathroom: Rebuilding Your Social Life With DI

Coyote's Gift for Decision Makers

Ghoul-Goo: Spooky S'mores You'll Die For

Echoes in the Mirror: Scrying and Self-Destruction Magick

Thread and Thorn: Stitching Spells from Rural Cloth

The Mogwai Mind: Building Untouchable Wealth from Small Ideas

Be Your Own Guide: Trust Your Inner Compass

Hormones in Chaos: The Endocrine Puzzle of Diabetes Insipidus

ChronoCleanse: Detox Your Biological Timeline

The Limb You Hide Is the One That Saves You

Leaves, Bones, and Whisper Spells

The Dinosaur Mindset: Prehistoric Tactics for Modern Wealth

Clawing Back Control: A Bastet Method for Boundaries and Empowerment

Samhain Codes of the Forgotten

Orange Alchemy: The Autumnal Spellbook

Monster Within, Master Without

The Sigil That Sleeps

Hearthcraft: Yule Hearth Sigils and Winter Warmth Spells

Temple of the Purring Moon: Rituals from Bastet's Lineage

When the Earth Remembers Your Footsteps

Food for Mood: Eat to Heal Depression, Not Just Survive It
Witch of the Kudzu Vine: Southern Pagan Wealth Secrets
The Invisible Diagnosis: Advocating for Yourself With DI
The Coffin's Lullaby: Sleep Magick and Nightmares as Portals
Ashes of the Will: Rituals for Erasing the Self
The Fracture Rite: Shattering the Magickal Core
Funeral Candles: The Art of Emo Flame Magick
The Black Grimoire: A Blank Ritual for Writing in Absence
Phantom Thirst: A Halloween Survival Guide for Diabetes Insipidus
The Hollow Crown: Emo Royalty and Magick of the Outcast King
Sandpainting for the Soul
Falling Into Balance: Using the Extra Hour to Recalibrate Life
100 Southern Superstitions That Still Work
The DI Child: A Parent's Guide to Raising Hydrated, Happy Kids
The Jungle of Shame: Escaping the Hidden Lab of Doubt
The Witch's Toast: S'mores Spells and Creepy Confections
The Hoodoo Pantry: Spells from the Mason Jar
The Immortal Fortune: Secret Wealth Lessons from Captain Jack Harkness
The Specter's Embrace: Magick for Channeling Ghostly Lovers
Grateful Waters: A Thanksgiving Survival Guide for Diabetes Insipidus
The Seizure Gospel
Harvestbind: Autumn Sigils and Samhain Spells
Doctor Who: The Algorithmic Awakening
Silent Nights, Steady Waters: A Christmas Survival Guide for Diabetes Insipidus
The Extra Hour Effect: How One Hour Can Transform Everything

Blade Between the Breaths

Running with the Mountain Shadows

Echoes of the Failed Experiment – Becoming a Living Legacy

Swamp Witches & River Ghosts: Real Southern Hauntings

Cornbread Prophecies: Magical Recipes from a Southern Table

Doctor Who: The Signal in the Star

Bloomcraft: Spring Sigils and Equinox Enchantments

Vanisher: How to Disappear from the Internet Without Losing Your Life

The Ultimate Christmas Cookie Cookbook

The Unbreakable Parent: How to Mentally Survive Raising Kids in a Broken World

Time Debt: How to Reclaim the Hours You Didn't Know You Lost

One Month, One Million: Unconventional Cash Creation Tactics

Doctor Who: The Cyber Conversion Protocol

Black Friday Frenzy: The Art of Finding Hidden Online Deals

The Grimoire Buried Under the Apple Tree

Digital Couponing Masterclass: Your Step-by-Step Guide to Black Friday Savings

The Fire Inside the Flint

Shadows on the Ceiling: The Emo Guide to Astral Magick

The Bone-Eaters Beneath Us

Black Friday Bundle Blueprint: Creating Irresistible Product Packages for Maximum Sales

Thirteen Nights of Unbinding

Doctor Who: Engines of Influence

Pumpkin Spice Alchemy: Recipes of Fire and Frost

When Raptor Met Rexy: Prehistoric Lessons in Wild Romance

Oblivion's Candle: Burn the Path Behind You

Campfire Curses and Chocolate: A Halloween S'mores Grimoire

The Wallet That Wasn't Mine: Breaking Free from Inherited Scarcity

The Cola Zodiac: What Your Fizz Says About Your Fate

Frostfire Fortune: Unlocking Winter's Hidden Prosperity

Signal Jamming: Detox Your Brain from Info Overload

The Dust of the Forgotten Rite

The Golden Cat Sigils: Drawing Power in Bastet's Name

Mud Magick: The Prosperity of Getting Dirty

Savory Spicefall: Beyond the Pumpkin Pie

Pumpkin Spice Apothecary Kitchen

The Pumpkin Spice Economy: Turning Trends into Billions

The Ember Veil: 13 Nights of Fire Magick

Financial Freeze: When Earning Triggers Panic

The Gingerbread Alchemist: Sweet Recipes with a Twist

Biosynth Power: Programming Yourself from Scratch

Echoes from the Talking Circle

Truffle Alchemy: Fungus of Fortune

Spores of Power: The Truffle Witch's Handbook

Doctor Who: The Tower That Speaks

The Mycelium Veil: Truffle Magick Unbound

Broke But Ashamed: Healing the Shame Wound of Debt

The Evergreen Mind: Growth Through Winter Stillness

The Black Veil Truffle Rite

The Voice Beneath Symbols

Witchlight on the Bayou: Swamp Spells for Sovereignty

I Grew Up Poor and Now I Sabotage My Success

The Lantern of Hollow Souls

Shutdown Survival: A Citizen's Guide to Thriving When Government Stops

When Abundance Feels Like a Threat: Healing the Hidden Fears of Enough

The Scarecrow Grimoire
Owls of the October Veil
Candlewax and Curses: A Halloween Spellbook
Excavating the Inner Fossil – Transforming Fossilized Thoughtforms into Tools of Power
The Yule Witch's Spellbook: Magick for the Holiday Season
Haunted Christmas: Ghost Stories for Winter Nights
The Christmas Survival Guide: Thriving Through the Chaos
The Bone Orchard Rites
Haunted Commerce: The Ghost in the Marketplace
When Money Triggers the Inner Child
Silent Night with the Silence: A Christmas Thriller
The Lightning Crown: Living and Leading Through Seizures
TARDIS Tidings: Festive Stories from the Whoniverse
Autumn Reset: Slowing Down Without Falling Behind
The Trillion Dollar Soul: Rewriting the Currency of Reality
Truffle Eclipse Magick
Micro-Manifestations: Quick Magick That Works
5-Minute Rituals for Busy Witches
The Marshmallow Massacre: Halloween Treats with a Sinister Twist
Blood and Blackberry Thorns
Magickal Mornings: Rituals for a Blessed Christmas Day
Embers of the All-Hallows Fire
The Pumpkin Market Collapse
The Hour You Gained: Transforming Time Into Power
The Chamber Must Be Sealed: Mastering the Power of Controlled Access
The Cursed Manuscript of Petosiris
The Festive Hearth: Creating Holiday Traditions
Darkness Rising: Thriving as Nights Grow Longer
Harvesting Time: Turning the Year's End Into Your New Beginning

Petosiris and the 13th Zodiac Key
Wagewound: When Paychecks Become Identity Prisons
Walls That Watch
The Silent Feast: Rituals of Power in the Longest Night
The Distortus Legacy : Becoming a Deformed King in a Perfect World
The Hollow Masks
The Gratitude Furnace: Forging Gold from Thanks
Feast of Inner Gold: Eating for Energy and Enlightenment
Haunted Commerce: The Season of Spending Spirits
Fear Bonds: How Panic Creates Profit
Black Friday E-Commerce Playbook: Sales Tactics to Skyrocket Your Holiday Revenue
Budgeting for Black Friday: A Holiday Savings Planner
Haunting the Harvest Moon
The Warrior's Water: Emergency Preparedness for People With DI
The First Sip of the Year: A New Year's Survival Guide for Diabetes Insipidus
Doctor Who: The Thirteenth Node
The Unseen Struggle: Mental Health, Anxiety, and Chronic Thirst
The Hearth's Hidden Ledger: Counting Energies as Currency
The Gift Alchemist: Turning Any Offering Into Gold
The Papyrus of the Bound Spirit
The Magick of Leftovers: Transmutation in the Fridge
Frost and Fortune: Christmas Wealthcraft for the Modern Magus
Last-Minute Gifts: Creative Ideas on a Budget
10 Secrets to Surviving Holiday Crowds
The Witch's Dow Jones
The Witches' Graveyard Shift
Pumpkin Sigils: Carving Rites for Midnight Power

The Secret Shopper's Black Friday Guide: How to Get Early Access and VIP Deals

Fever in the Foundation

The Neuralyzer Reset: Reprogram Your Morning Routine

Lightning Lessons of the White Painted Woman

The Enchanted Snowflake

The Magic Sip: Surviving Disney Parks with Diabetes Insipidus

The One Who Draws Through You

Santa's Secrets: A Magical Holiday Planner

Silent Bells, Loud Miracles: Self-Help for the Season of Stillness

The Sugar Spell Codex: Confectionary Magick of Christmas

Autumn Hexcraft: Fallen Leaves, Fallen Barriers

Sleep Like a Fortress: Build a Life Where Insomnia Can't Survive

Nowhere Was Ever Home

Christmas Under the Stars: A Celestial Holiday Guide

Rentproof: How to Never Be Evicted Again

Workless: Escape the 9-5 Without Being Broke

The Gilded Gift: A Wealth Altar for Christmas Morning

The Black Friday Grimoire

The Hollowing: Ceremonies of Spiritual Collapse

Doctor Who: The Nameless Signal

Where the Eagle Hides His Courage

The Dwarf Tyrant's Ascent: Claiming Power in a World of Giants

The Currency of the Dead: Trading with Spectral Bankers

The Icebound Witch: Survival and Magick in the Cold

The Emergency Money Mind: Constant Crisis, Zero Calm

Thirst & Roses: A Valentine's Survival Guide for Diabetes Insipidus

Springing Into Clarity: Mastering the Energy Shift of Daylight Saving

Speed of the Nanotyrant: Agile Strategies for Life's Hunt

The 90-Day Reset: A Science-Backed Guide to Reinvent Yourself Before the New Year

The Coil of Thorns

Timegates Unleashed

Dopamine Fasting 2.0: Rewiring Your Brain in a World of Overstimulation

The Nanotyrannus Mutation: Embracing Your Differentiated Form

Unwritten January: How to Use the Blank Page of the Year to Re-Author Your Life

Feast of the Forgotten Spirits: Ancestor Magick for the Holidays

The Burnout Codex: A System for Thriving Beyond Stress

I Don't Deserve to Have Money

When the King Doesn't See You: The Shadow Predator's Guide

The Reset Ritual :A Guide to Shedding Last Year's Weight—Emotional and Physical—by Spring Cleaning Your Soul

Calendar Alchemy: Learn to Bend Time and Productivity around Your Natural Rhythms

The Mirror Contract: A One-Sentence Agreement with Yourself that Unlocks Real Change

The Nile Formula: Sacred Flow for Millionaire Minds

Forward Momentum: Productivity Rituals for the Lost Hour

Harvest Gold: Wealth Magick of Pumpkin Spice Commerce

The Magick of Christmas Lights: Illuminating Holiday Rituals

Cranberry Crown: Royal Self-Worth through Ritual Meals

Petosiris and the Worms of the Feathered Throne

The Evergreen Equation: Self-Help for Sustained Growth

The Rain Will Wash Us Away: Emo Weather Magick

Snowlight Shadows: Magick Under Frozen Stars

Doctor Who: Merger of Empires

The Light Within the Feast: Magickal Wealth of Yuletide Flame

Momentum Machines: Small Habits Designed to Snowball into Unstoppable Forward Motion

Calm Spells: Magickal Solutions for Anxiety Relief

Santa's Final List: The Naughty Never Leave

The Mystic's Guide to Banishing Worry

The Silence Dividend: Turning Quiet Mornings into Compounding Growth All Year

Charmed Stillness: Rituals to Ease the Mind

Blood Spiral Ascension

The Vanishing Heart Invocation

Crystal Calm: Harnessing Stones for Anxiety

The Nano Tyrant Code: Strength in the Small Predator

The Energy Ledger: Accounting Methods for Vitality, Not Just Money

Snowglobe Mindset: Shake Up Your Thoughts, Settle Into Peace

The Weight of the Feather: Anubis's Codes for Soul Balance

Pocket Peppermint Power: Tiny Rituals for Big Holiday Energy

Shadowkeeper of the Golden Jackal: Anubis's Path to Energetic Protection

The Witch's Breath: Anxiety Relief Through Magickal Breathing

The Tiny Ember: Pocket Motivation for Cold Days

Stocking Sorcery: Mini Spells for Holiday Luck and Prosperity

Warm Hands, Steady Heart: Micro Grounding for Winter Anxiety

The Jackal's Lantern: Guide-Lights for Walking the Dark Path

Anubis's Silent Steps: Rituals for Stealth, Peace & Emotional Quiet

The Bonewake Protocol

Extinction-Proof: How to Outlive Trends, Trauma, and Time

The Fourth Doctor: The Eccentric Wanderer

The Second Doctor: Chaos and Charm in the TARDIS (Patrick Troughton, 1966–1969)

The Third Doctor: Earthbound Defender of Time (Jon Pertwee, 1970–1974)

The First Doctor: Genesis of the Time Lord (William Hartnell, 1963–1966)

The Fourth Doctor: The Eccentric Wanderer ***(Tom Baker, 1974–1981)***

The Fifth Doctor: Elegance and Empathy (Peter Davison, 1982–1984)

The Sixth Doctor: A Kaleidoscope of Conflict (Colin Baker, 1984–1986)

The Seventh Doctor: The Strategist of Shadows (Sylvester McCoy, 1987–1989)

The Eighth Doctor: A Time Lord's Renaissance (Paul McGann, 1996)

The War Doctor: A Time Lord's Burden (John Hurt, 2013)

The Ninth Doctor: The Healer of Worlds
(Christopher Eccleston, 2005)

The Tenth Doctor: The Lonely Hero (David Tennant, 2005–2010)

The Eleventh Doctor: The Madman in a Box (Matt Smith, 2010–2013)

The Twelfth Doctor: The Rebel with a Cause (Peter Capaldi, 2013–2017)

The Thirteenth Doctor: Breaking the Mold
(Jodie Whittaker, 2017–2022)

The Fourteenth Doctor: A New Beginning (David Tennant, 2022–2023)

The Fifteenth Doctor: Rewriting the Stars
(Ncuti Gatwa, 2023–2025)

Santa's Shortcut to Success: Micro Habits for a Better New Year

The Midnight Cocoa Manifesto: Comfort Rituals for Hard Nights

Why I Can't Save: Trauma Blocks to Financial Planning

Dino Brain, Mega Goals: Rewire Yourself for Savage Success.

Jurassic Profit: Unearth Your Inner Millionaire Fossil

Scales & Softness: Dating with Dino Heart

Carnotaurus Dreams.

Red Willow Thinking.

Reindeer Resilience: How to Keep Going When You're Exhausted

Candlewick Courage: Lighting Strength in Dark Seasons.

Elf-Mode Focus: Fast Attention Fixes for Busy Seasons

Futureproof Feelings: Emotional Skill-Building for Resilience No Matter What the New Year Brings

The 90-Day Rewire: Transform Your Neural Pathways Before Spring Blooms

Jolly Rich: Christmas Micro-Money Magick for Fast Prosperity.

Gingerbread Gratitude: Mini Practices for a Happier Holiday

Trauma-Spending: When Money Becomes a Drug

Goal Skeletons: Build Minimalist Frameworks for Resolutions That Last

The Snarl Strategy: Growling Back at a World That Silenced You

The Hourglass Reset: Reclaiming What the Clock Took

Yule Claw: Dino Rites of Light in the Darkness

Sacred Circles: Grounding Rituals for Anxious Souls

Clockstopper's Gut: Rebuilding the Core of Time

Winterfire Drive: Harness the Cold Season's Stillness to Ignite Deep Motivation

The 5-Minute Productivity Hack: Small Steps to Big Results

Light Ascending: A Self-Help Guide to Longer Days

Inner Economy: Trade Self-Doubt for Confidence Like a High-Value Currency

Simple Success: Decluttering Your Life for Better Results

The Resilient Mind: Thriving in Tough Times

The 2026 Playbook: Mastering the Year Ahead

The Spring Sleep Solution: Conquering Fatigue After Time Change.

The Hormonal Compass: Navigate Back to Your Youth

Golden Vision: Eating for Your Eye Color with the Power of Ghee

Lionhearted Love: Strength in Relationships

MiB Mindset: Think Like a Cosmic Agent

The Ladder of Small Wins: Climb Out of Stagnation by Stacking Micro-Victories

The Momentum Hour: Gaining More in Less Time.

The Year of You: A Self-Help Blueprint for Unapologetic Self-Ownership

The Dust That Watches You Back.

The Astral Parent

Shadow of the King: The Nanotyrannus Parable

Tiny Tidings of Triumph: Small Wins That Change Your Life

Dwarf Tyrant Rising: When You're the One They Overlook

The Bank Account Mirror: Healing How You See Yourself Through Money

Cretaceous Black

When Love Costs Too Much: Romantic Triggers and Financial Wounds

Dream-Eater's Guide to Wealth

Unzipped Reality: The Jacket That Opens Portals

The Power of No: How to Set Boundaries and Get Rich

Keeper of the Desert Veil: Anubis's Teachings on Illusion & Truth

Redacted Stargates: Stories the SGC Buried

The Clock That Dripped Time

Doctor Who: The Silent Acquisition

Hairline Manifestation: Unlocking Power at the Edge of Thought

Cash-Eater Crickets: How Insects Predict Economic Collapse

Dead Pet Whisperer: Grief Alchemy from the Other Side

The Love Algorithm Is Broken: Hack Romance Before It Hacks You

The Rite of the 8-Limbed Seal

Melt the Moon: A Fire Ritual to Reshape Emotion

Venomous Miracles: Healing Through the Poison Path

Wealth Without Water: The Post-Aquatic Rich Life

The Butterfly Betrayal: When Change Turns on You

The Quiet Upgrade: How Humans Are Secretly Rebuilding Themselves Without Asking Permission

Nobody Taught Us This: The Missing Human Manual for Money, Energy, and Self-Respect

You Were Never Broken: Why Most People Are Reacting Normally to an Unstable World

After the Noise Ends: How Humans Reset When the World Finally Goes Quiet

The Month That Tells the Truth: Why January Reveals What the Rest of the Year Hides

Tremors Party Unleashed: The Ultimate Guide to a Graboids Birthday Bash

Cold Start Human: Rebooting Motivation Without Forcing Momentum

The Year that doesn't start until they say

Love Without Performance: What Connection Looks Like When No One Is Watching

February Is a Mirror: What Love Exposes About You

How We Learned Love Wrong: Uninstalling Cultural Myths About Connection

You Are Not Too Much: Why Needing Love Is Not a Flaw

The Crooked Fence Covenant: Backwoods Boundaries and Witch Wealth

The Day That Keeps Repeating: Why Your Life Feels Stuck—and How to Shift It Gently

Nothing Changes Until Something Softens: Escaping Repetition Without Violence to Yourself

Same Life, Different Ending: How Tiny Choices Rewrite Repetition

The Loop Isn't Punishment: Why You're Being Asked to Learn, Not Suffer

Panic at the Register: Retail Anxiety and Public Shame

The Secret Formula to Becoming an Influencer in 90 Days

The New Rich: How to Retire by 35

Digital Nomad Secrets: How to Travel the World and Make Millions

Burn Your Waiting Room: Escape the Delay Spiral

Strapped for Pleasure: A Complete Guide to Pegging and Strap-On Play

Locked in Desire: A Guide to Chastity Play and Intimate Control

Burrowing into History: Groundhog Day Through the Ages

The Shadow Forecast: The Science of Groundhog Day

Choice Cascades: How One Decision in January Sets Ripples for the Whole Year

The Anti-Anxiety Blueprint: Mastering Fear and Stress for Success

The Ancestral Path of the Jackal Priest

Winterborn Titans: Giants of Ice and Stone

The Extinction Spire

The Emotion That Made Me Millions

Delete Their Voice: Become Unreachable

The Frostbound Mysteries: Mythical Beings of January's Chill

The Roar Within: Unlocking Your Potential

From Burrow to Sky: Groundhog Day Explained

The Boogey Book: Festive Ward-Off Edition

Fooled Ya! The Psychology Behind Great Pranks

April Fools' Alchemy: Transforming Everyday Items into Pranks

Anchor Habits: Root Yourself in Unshakable Routines That Endure Seasonal Change

Emerald Waters: A St. Patrick's Day Survival Guide for Diabetes Insipidus

The Groundhog's Legacy: Myths, Legends, and Facts

Six Weeks of Mystery: The Truth Behind Groundhog Day

The Upgrade Mind: Tech-Like Patches and Updates for Your Mental Operating System

Moon Blood, Star Flesh: Embracing Your Hybrid Nature

Groundhog Lore and Legend: A Complete Guide

You Are the Lie They Can't Kill

Download a Different Reality

The Quiet Advantage: Winning Without Announcing Yourself

A Year of Gratitude: Unlocking Joy

Touch Grass: A Pagan Reset for a Burned-Out Digital World

Cold Start Wealth: Building Financial Power from a Standing Still Point

Astrology Without Fate: Using Cycles Without Surrendering Control

The Future is Remote: Work Less, Earn More, Live Anywhere

Harvest of Silence

The Algorithm Knows Your Name
April Fools' Day for Introverts
Soft Power Systems: Influence That Doesn't Exhaust You
Practical Magick for Real Life: Focus, Intent, and Follow-Through
January Is a Lie: Designing Momentum Without the Calendar
Universal Flow: Managing DI in High-Energy Theme Parks
Electric Allure: Exploring Erotic Electro-Play
The Masked Embrace: Exploring Sensory Deprivation
The Ultimate April Fools' Survival Guide
Splashproof Survival: Waterparks & Wave Pools with DI
Agile Predator, Still King: Crafting Your Speed in a World That Celebrates Size
The Shadow Feast: Groundhog Day's Sinister Side
The Bug's Business Model
Edge of Bliss: Mastering the Art of Tease and Denial
Midnight Alchemy: Rituals for Transformation Between the Old Year and the New
Punxsutawney Bloodlines: A Groundhog Day Horror
The Burrower: Groundhog Day's Darkest Secrets
Buried Alive: A Groundhog Day Horror Story
Blood Moon Markets: The Witch's Guide to Wealth Magick
The Groundhog's Shadow: What It Means for the World
Seasonal Shadows: The Groundhog Day Phenomenon
The Shadow's Curse: A Groundhog Day Horror Tale
Punxsutawney Revealed: A Guide to Groundhog Day
Safari Hydration: Zoo & Wildlife Park Survival for DI
The Foolproof Prank Planner
***Latex Lust: Embracing Fetish Fashion* is a sophisticated**
Whip & Whisper: The Dynamics of Impact Play
The Shadow Burrow Chronicles: Horror Beneath the Ground
Frozen Shadows: A Groundhog Day Thriller
The Groundhog's Revenge: A February Nightmare

Burrow of the Damned
Everyday Enchantment: Magickal Practices for Modern Living
Budget Bliss: The Easy Path to Financial Freedom
Six More Weeks of Terror
The Oxygen Debt
The Ice Veil: Mystical Beasts of January's Shadows
Roots That Remember
Polar Myths: Creatures of the Icy Abyss
The Marginalia Covenant
AI and the Occult: Digital Spirits, Sigils, and Cyber-Witchcraft
Roleplay Realms: Crafting Fantasies and Scenes
The Last Clean River
Lover in the Shadows: A Groundhog Day Tale
Buried Hearts: A Groundhog Day Gothic Romance
Anubis Wept for Petosiris
The Lantern Knows Your Name
Rituals of the Last Shadow
The Bell That Rings for No One
Shadows of Love and Death
The Groundhog's Bride: A Dark Valentine's Tale
Frozen Kisses: A Horror Romance for Groundhog Day
The Creative Spark: Igniting Your Passion Projects
From Cub to King: A Journey of Transformation
Six Weeks to Midnight: A Groundhog Day Romance
Tide of the Unclean
Burrow of Desire: A Groundhog Day Paranormal Romance
The Shadow Magick Almanac: Harnessing Groundhog Day Energies
AI for Emo Influencers: Growing an Online Following Without the Anxiety
AI for the Melancholy Millionaire: Making Money Without Social Interaction

Winter's Grip: A Horror Romance Beneath the Frost
Shadowed Hearts: A Love Buried in Winter's Chill
The Shadow Lover: A Groundhog Day Gothic Love Story
Beneath the Burrow: A Groundhog Day Thriller
The Punxsutawney Conspiracy
The Crimson Pact: Emo Blood Oath Magick
The Shadows of Gallifrey: A Doctor Who Horror Collection
Whispers in the Vortex: Chilling Tales from the TARDIS
AI Ghostwriting for Emo Souls: How to Make Money Writing Without Trying
The Anti-Social Emo's Guide to AI-Powered Freelancing
Emo AI Therapy: Talking to Robots When Humans Suck
Cry & Collect: AI-Powered Passive Income for Emos
The Weeping Angel Chronicles: A Collection of Terror
Dating Without the Mask
The Clockwork Menace: Horror Stories from the Future
Tender Doesn't Mean Weak
Not a Burden, Not a Bonus
Dalek Nightmares: Stories of Ultimate Extermination
The Empty Child's Curse: Tales of Horror and Fear
The TARDIS Ghost Files: Hauntings Across the Universe
Soft Armor, Open Heart
Chosen Gently
Love That Doesn't Rush You
Financial Gaslighting: When You're Made to Feel Crazy About Money.
After the Bees Went Silent
The Soil Knows Your Name
The Quantum Magick Codex: Unlocking the Hidden Laws of Reality
The Gingerbread Golem's Awakening: A Tale of Sweet Revenge

The Gingerbread Golem Chronicles: Guardians of Frost Hollow

The Power of Focus: Eliminate Distractions, Achieve Greatness

Sacred Submission: The Dynamics of D/s Relationships

The Magick of Numbers: Unlocking the Hidden Codes of the Universe

Blood and Bones: The Ancient Magick of Life and Death

Doctor Who: The Collapse Dividend

Thesis of the Unremembered

Desired as You Are

The Energy Budget of Love

Romancing Your Potential: The Love Month Growth Guide

Seen, Not Studied

Screams from the Void: Horror Stories Inspired by Doctor Who

The Silence Is Watching: A Collection of Dread

Under the Floorboards

The House of Feathers and Fangs

Emperor Bones, Hollow Crown

Goreglyphs of the Boiling Deep

The Coven That Screamed Back

The Stacks That Breathe

Love That Adapts

Nightmares on Gallifrey: Frights from the Doctor Who Universe

Apache Ways to Heal Powerfully

Belos Left No Corpses

The Algorithm Hates You (Good.)

Starve the Soul, Feed the Flame

Romance Without Apology

The Carbon Illusion

Your Nervous System is Your GPS

Where Rest Learns Your Name: Six Gentle Bedtime Stories for Minds That Work Differently
Soft Armor for Tender Nights: Six 5-Minute Bedtime Stories for Hearts That Have Been Hurt
Paws of Night, Path of Stars: Six 5-Minute Bedtime Stories Guided by Bastet and Anubis
When the Mind Needs a Lamp: Six 5-Minute Bedtime Stories for Gentle Mental Health Care
Imbolc Roar: Awakening the Dino Flame
The Titan Never Died
Witchflesh Harvest
Become the Thought They Can't Unsee
Golden Threads: The Sensuality of Body Worship
Chains of Desire: Exploring the Beauty of Restraint
Glyphs Written in Organs
Living Below the Line
Palismen Don't Scream—Until They Do
The Boiling Isles Devour the Weak
Hexside Anatomy Lab
Philip Wittebane and the First Body
Money PTSD: When Trauma Hijacks Your Finances
Brother, Bone, and Betrayal
Lipstick Like a Weapon: A Goth Girl's Guide to Emotional Dominance, Boundaries, and Quiet Intimidation
The Scar Is the Portal
Don't Grow—Mutate
Built from Breakdown: The Collapse Code
The Collector's First Lesson
Glyph Failure Syndrome
Philip Wittebane and the Discipline of Lies
The Making of Belos
Flesh Does Not Belong
The Golden Guard Prototypes

Coven Marks as Control Wounds
The Voice Belos Invented
The Boogeyman Within: Shadow Work for Personal Transformation
The Energy Edge: Reclaiming Your Power
Mindful March: A Quick Guide to Intentional Living
Love on Autopilot: Rekindle Your Relationship Instantly
Spring Renewal: Refresh Your Mindset Before the Equinox
Velvet Control: The Subtle Art of Erotic Choking
Erotic Shadows: Playing with Voyeurism and Exhibitionism
The Green Pulse Awakens
Equinox Bones
Immortality Is a Disease
Cold-Blooded Focus
The Invasive Advantage
The Lonely Assassin's Love: A Weeping Angel Romance
Philip Is Still Inside
Become the Signal That Replaces the Noise
When the Soil Says Yes
Shedding What No Longer Protects You
The Shadow Key: Unlocking the Power of Your Dark Self
The Enchanted Chocolate Rituals: Magickal Recipes for Love & Wealth
Love in the Vortex: A Doctor Who Horror Romance
Grimwalker Number Seventeen
The Boy Who Woke Again
Sad Girls Don't Beg: Reclaiming Self-Worth When Melancholy Is Mistaken for Weakness
Raising Pagan Children in a Non-Pagan World
The Pagan Homeschool Exit Strategy
Protecting Childhood While Preparing for Adulthood
Curriculum for the Dead
Too Much for Who? Reclaiming the Power of Intensity

Your Nervous System Is the Algorithm
Memories That Don't Belong to Him
The Golden Guard Template
Time-Locked Hearts: A Gallifreyan Gothic Romance
Ostara's Hatchlings: Fertile Dino Magick
The Dalek's Heart: A Tale of Forbidden Love
The Jackal's Final Game
Where Wild Magic Took My Brother
Where Love Meets Reality
Volume Without Apology
The Mind of Stillness: Petosiris's Hidden Teachings on Power
Doctor Who: The Final Shareholder Meeting
The Archive of Unfinished Lives
AI for Emo Musicians: Automating Your Sad Soundtracks
AI-Generated Emo Art: Selling Melancholy in Digital Form
Ashes Where the Cathedral Slept
The Monarch of Splintered Wings
People-Pleasing Is a Survival Strategy Past Its Expiration Date
Velvet Carnage Covenant
The Intensity Advantage
Attention Is a Finite Resource—You're Overspending It
Emotional Debt Compounds Faster Than Money
The Siege of Thornlit Graves
When the Bone King Wept Black
Comfort Is the Most Expensive Addiction
The AI Gothpreneur: Building a Business Without Any Social Interaction
AI & Tarot: Emo Divination for the Digital Age
Sad AI Aesthetics: Emo Branding & Personal Style
Black Sails Over a Dying Sun
The Crimson Parliament of Wolves
Cathedral of Veins and Thunder
The Orchard of Hanging Saints

The Self-Discovery Path: Find Your True Purpose
You Were Taught to Self-Sabotage Politely
Chrysalis Debt: Reborn into Wealth
Empire of Teeth and Perfume
The Devourer's Bride of Iron Mist
The Dormitory with No Windows
Built Larger Than the Room
The Silence Between Wings
The Manuscript That Grades You
The Librarian Who Refused to Die
Footnotes for a Burning Campus
The Thornblood Accord
The Paranormal Files: True Encounters with Ghosts, Aliens, and the Unexplained
Warfare in the Temple of Shattered Constellations
The Crow's Codex: Unlocking the Secrets of the Black-Winged Messengers
Purring Boundaries: Bastet's Guide to Raising Fierce Children
The Arcane Wealth Formula: Spellcasting for Infinite Abundance
The Celestial Spellbook: Harnessing Planetary Magick for Power and Fortune
Silk Shrouds of the Frostbound Wilds
Windtalker: The Hill Witch's Guide to Whisper Magick
The Doctrine of Psyence: Knowledge Beyond the Veil
The Bone Sovereign's Final War Chant
The Abyssal Altar of Salt and Silver
The Lantern Wilds That Devoured Lovers
The Court of the Sable Scar
Wax & Whispers: The Art of Candle Play
The Billionaire's Blueprint: Unlocking Wealth Through Action

The Cleansing Flow: Unlocking Wellness with Enema Therapy

Seasonal Gratitude: How to Thrive Before Spring

Beyond the Closet Door: Unlocking Your Full Potential by Embracing Fear

The War-Bound Crown

Eternity With Teeth

The Observer Is the Spell: Reality as Psychic Architecture

Mis-Classified Monster: Redefine Yourself

Claws Without Cruelty: The Bastet Discipline Method

Claws Without Cruelty: The Bastet Discipline Method

Temple Mothers: Parenting in the Spirit of the Sacred Cat

The Sixth Extinction You Can Stop

Ticket to the Unseen

The Basement Doesn't Stay Shut

Exhibit of Moving Bones

The Creek That Brings Things Back

No-Exit Hallway

The Tourist Who Knew Their Names

The Limestone Choir

The Room That Remembers Pain

Briar Hollow's Missing Hour

The Gift Shop of Cursed Souvenirs

The Stag in the Ceiling

Two Journals, One Lie

The Museum Eats Its Own Map

The Other Side Leaves Footprints

The Town That Forgets Faces

The Limestone Mouth

The Curator's Ledger of Regrets

The Portrait That Bleeds Tomorrow

The Visitor in Maeve's Voice

The Artifact That Wants to Be Worn

Briar Hollow's Second Sky
The Basement Opens in a Dream
Taxidermy That Isn't Dead
The Rift Key Wedding Ring
The Engine Under Limestone
The Town Under Pressure
Regret Is a Doorway
Boundary Law
The Bunker Beneath Briar Hollow
Concrete Cannot Keep It Out
Gravity Pockets
The Woman in the Static
The Rift Breathes.
Bone of the Threshold
The Cost of Return
The First Crossing
The Woman Who Came Back Wrong
Tethered Heart
The Heir Clause
Severance Geometry
The Witch's Shadow
After the Snap
THE LAND REMEMBERS
The Watchers in the Trees
Museum Under Surveillance
The Creek That Splits
The Line of Antlers
the beacon year
The First Wendigo Tracks
Hunger in the Pines
The Chupacabra Flock
Teeth in the Roof
Ghosts of the Overlap

The Double in the Creek
Forbidden Fruit: Kink and Food Play

www.ingramcontent.com/pod-product-compliance
Lightning Source LLC
LaVergne TN
LVHW022005200926
848481LV00007B/2235

* 9 7 9 8 2 9 5 6 8 8 4 0 9 *